CNA EXAM PREP

Volume 2

2nd Edition

Nurse Assistant Practice Test Questions

Jane John-Nwankwo RN, MSN

CNA EXAM PREP: Nurse Assistant Practice Test Questions

Volume 2

2nd Edition

ISBN-13: 978-1505919554

ISBN-10: 150591955X

Printed in the United States of America.

This book can be purchased at
www.djngbooks.org   www.janejohn-nwankwo.com

Dedication

Dedicated to my soul mate, John Nwankwo Ph.D who gave me all the support to publish this book

OTHER TITLES FROM THE SAME AUTHOR:

1. Work At Home Jobs For Nurses & Other Healthcare Professionals

2. Nurses' Romance Series

3. Hightime you made a move! An inspirational and motivational book

4. Patient Care Technician Exam Review Questions: PCT Test Prep

5. Design Your Own Methods To Navigate

6. EKG Technician Study Guide

7. BLS for Healthcare Providers Student Manual

8. Phlebotomy Test Prep Vol 1, 2, & 3

9. The Home Health Aide Textbook

10. Accept Challenges

11. CNA Study Guide

And Many More Books

Visit www.healthcarepracticetest.com

www.janejohn-nwankwo.com

www.bookaspeakernow.com

www.djngbooks.org

Have you bought these books?

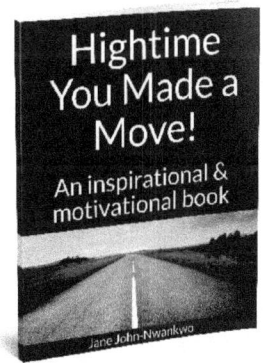

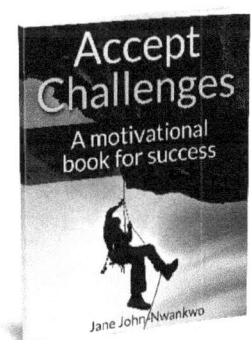

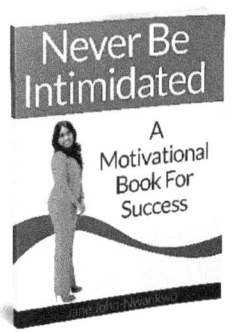

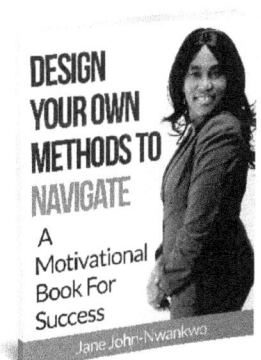

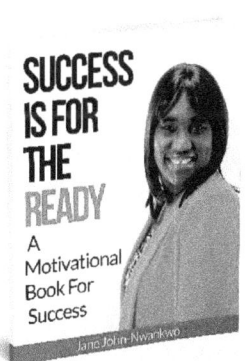

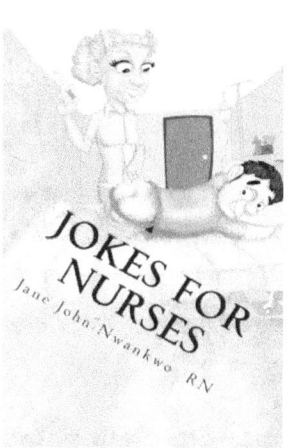

Buy these books at www.janejohn-nwankwo.com
www.djngbooks.org

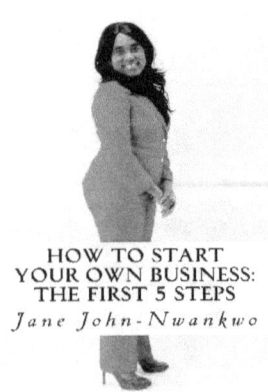

HOW TO START
YOUR OWN BUSINESS:
THE FIRST 5 STEPS
Jane John-Nwankwo

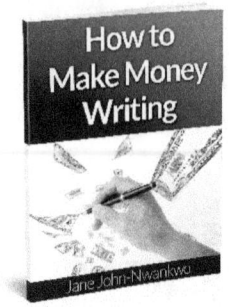

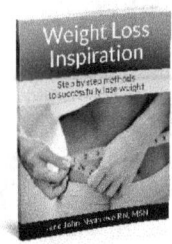

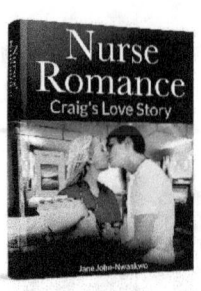

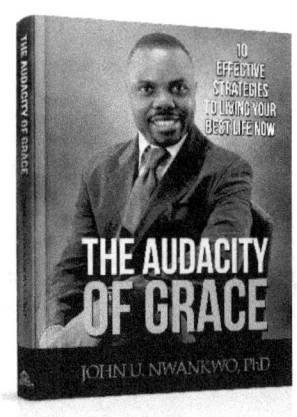

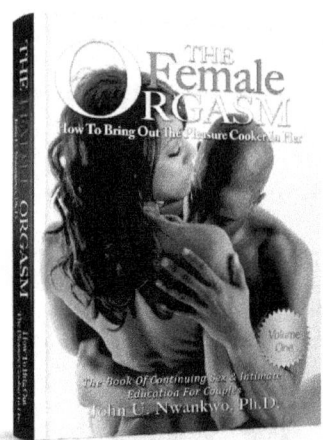

Buy these books at www.janejohn-nwankwo.com
www.djngbooks.org

TABLE OF CONTENTS

1. _____ are people or organizations paying for health care services

   A. Payers

   B. Providers

   C. Facilities

2. LTC mean

   A. Length of care

   B. Length of cure

   C. Long term care

3. When an individual is expected to die from an illness, it is referred to as a

   A. Terminal illness

   B. Acute illness

   C. Chronic illness

4. Most conditions seen in long term care facilities are chronic

   A. True

   B. False

5. _____ care is given in hospitals and ambulatory surgical centers.

   A. Acute care

   B. Home healthcare

   C. Adult daycare

6. Which of the following care can be given in a hospital or in a long-term care facility?

   A. Hospice care

B. Home Health care

C. Sub-acute care

7. After removing gloves, you are not required to wash your hands.

A. True

B. False

8. Which of the following care is usually for 24 hours?

A. Out-patient care

B. Skilled Care

9. Daily personal care tasks are called

A. Active daily living

B. Activities in daily living

C. Activities of daily living (ADLs)

10. A thin tube inserted into the body that is used to drain fluids or inject fluid is

A. Drainage

B. Catheter

C. Intravenous

11. Which one of the following is defined as the loss of mental abilities, such as thinking, remembering, reasoning, and communicating?

A. Dementia

B. Stroke

C. Acute coronary syndrome

12. What does "p" mean in PASS while operating a fire extinguisher?

A. Pin

B. Pull

    C. Point

13. _____ is a method, or way of doing something

    A. Procedure

    B. Policy

    C. Rules

14. Caucasian women make up a high percentage of residents in long term care facilities

    A. True

    B. False

15. Nursing assistants should accept money and gifts from residents

    A. True

    B. False

16. To cite means to

    A. Review a problem though a survey

    B. Find a problem through survey

    C. Create a problem through a survey

17. _____ is an independent not-for-profit organization that evaluates and accredits healthcare organizations.

    A. OSHA

    B. Health Care Finance Administration (HCFA)

    C. Joint Commission on Accreditation of Healthcare Organization(JCAHO)

18. Medicare and Medicaid pay long-term care facilities a fixed amount for services

    A. True

    B. False

19. Tuberculosis is _____transmitted

    A. Blood-borne

B. Airborne

C. contact

20. People who live in long term care facilities are usually called

   A. Clients

   B. Residents

C. Patients

SECTION TWO

Match the following

1. CNA _____   A. Direct plan activities for residents to help them socialize and stay physically and mentally active.

2. RN _____   B. Determines residents' needs and helps get them support services such as counseling.

3. LPN/LVN _____   C. Creates diets for resident with specials needs

4. MD/DO _____   D. Help with speech and swallowing problems

5. PT _____   E. Helps residents learn to compensate for disabilities

6. OT _____   F. Evaluates a person and develops a treatment plan to increase movement, improve circulation, promote healing

7. SLP ___   G. Diagnose disease or disability and prescribe treatment

8. RD ___   H. Licensed professional who has completed one to two years of education

9. MSW ___   I. Licensed professional who has completed two to four years of education

10. Activity Director ___   J. Performs delegated tasks such as taking vital signs, provides routine personal care, such as bathing residents and helping with toileting.

11. Professionalism means

    A. How you behave when you are on the job

    B. Having to do with work or a job

    C. Being late to work

12. Nursing assistants must be conscientious about documenting observations and procedures

    A. True

    B. False

13. _____ is the ability to understand what is proper and appropriate when dealing with others

    A. Sympathy

    B. Tact

    C. Empathy

Match the following

14. Compassionate ____   A. Put aside your opinions and see each resident as an individual who needs your care

15. Empathy ____   B. Give each resident the same quality care regardless of age, gender, race, ethnicity or condition

16. Sympathy _____   C. Valuing other individuality

17. Conscientious ___   D. Must make and keep commitments

18. Dependable _____   E. Always try to do their best

19. Respectful _____   F. Sharing in the feelings and difficulties of others

20. Unprejudiced _____   G. Entering into feeling of others

21. Tolerant _____   H. Being caring concerned, considerate, empathetic and understanding

22. Which of the following is not included in personal grooming habits

    A. Dressing neatly in a uniform that is washed and ironed

    B. Keep fingernails short, smooth and clean

    C. Wearing little or no makeup

    D. None of the above

23. The chain of command describes the line of authority and helps ensure that the resident receive proper care

    A. True

    B. False

24. _____ defines the things you are allowed to do and how to do them correctly.

    A. Scope of practice

    B. Unprejudiced

    C. Compassionate

    D. Tolerant

Match the following

25. Diagnosis _____   A. A careful examination to see if the goals are being met

26. Planning _____   B. Putting the care plan into action

27. Implementation ____   C. Setting goals and creating a care plan

28. Evaluation _____   D. Identifying the health problems after looking at all the resident's
    needs

29. Plan ahead _____   E. Identifying the most important things to get done

30. Prioritize _____   F. Best way to help manage your time better

SECTION THREE

1. The knowledge of right and wrong is

   A. Laws

   B. Rules

   C. Ethics

2. _____ are usually based on ethics

   A. Laws

   B. Rules

   C. Abuse

3. Behaving ethically and following the law applies to all healthcare providers.

   A. True

   B. False

4. _____ set minimum standards for nursing assistant training

   A. OSHA

   B. OBRA

   C. MDS

5. The _____ is a detailed form with guidelines for assessing residents

   A. OBRA

   B. MDS

   C. OSHA

6. Residents' rights include which of the following

   A. The right to make independent choices

   B. The right to participate in their own care

C. The right to privacy and confidentiality

D. All of the above

7. _____ is the process by which a person, with the help of a doctor makes decisions about his or her healthcare after sufficient information.

A. Living will

B. Informed consent

C. Power of attorney

8. Which of the following is a national non-profit organization founded in 1975 to protect the rights, safety and dignity of long-term care residents

A. Omnibus Budget Reconciliation Act(OBRA)

B. Joint Commission on Accreditation of Healthcare Organization(JCAHO)

C. The National Citizens' Coalition for Nursing Home Reform (NCCNHR)

Match the following

9. Neglect ____   A. another tool that help medical providers honor wishes about care

10. Active Neglect ____ B. Medical procedures to restart the heart and breathing

11. Passive Neglect __   C. A signed dated and witness paper

12. Negligence ____   D. Takes effect while the person is still living

13. Malpractice ____   E. Legal documents that allow people to choose what medical care they wish to have...

14. Abuse ____   F. Any unwelcome sexual advance behavior that creates an offensive working environment

15. Involuntary Seclusion __ G. Separating a person from others against the persons will

16. Sexual Harassment ____ H. Purposely causing Physical, mental or emotional pain or injury to someone

17. Advanced directives ____ I. Occurs when a person is injured due to professional misconduct through negligence

18. Living will ____   J. The failure to act to provide the proper care for a resident that result in unintended injury

19. Durable power of attorney ___ K. Unintentionally harming a person physically or by failing to provide care

20. Do-not-resuscitate (DNR) ___ L. Purposely harming a person by failing to provide needed care.

21. Cardiopulmonary resuscitation (CPR) ____ M. Harming a person physically or emotionally by failing to provide needed care

22. _____ are people who are legally required to report suspected or observed abuse or neglect

    A. Mandatory reporters

    B. News reported

    C. Mandated reporters

23. Which of the following is assigned by law as the legal advocate for residents

    A. Protected health information (PHI)

    B. Confidentiality

    C. Ombudsman

24. HIPAA means to

    A. Share private information with family members

    B. Keep patient information private

    C. Gives information to the public

25. Only people who give care or process records, should have access to protected health information

    A. True

    B. False

SECTION FOUR

1. _____ is the process of exchanging information with others

   A. Compassionate

   B. Sympathy

   C. Communication

2. The communication process consists of which of the following

   A. Sender, receiver and feedback

   B. Signs, symbols and drawings

   C. Drawings, receiver, sender

3. Verbal communication involves the use of words or sounds, spoken or written

   A. True

   B. False

4. Body language often speaks as words

   A. True

   B. False

5. _____ is the way we communicate without using words

   A. Culture

   B. Nonverbal communication

   C. Verbal communication

6. A _____ is a system of learned behaviors, practiced by a group of people

   A. Cultural diversity

   B. Culture

   C. Bias

7. Positive responses to cultural diversity include which of the following

   A. Acceptance and knowledge

   B. Bias and knowledge

   C. None of these

8. Which of the following are barriers to communication

   A. Resident is difficult to understand

   B. Advice is given

   C. Resident cannot hear you

   D. All of the above

9. All of the following are ways to make communication accurate except

   A. Giving advice

   B. Let some pauses happen

   C. Ask for more

10. When helping residents, do not talk to other staff

    A. True

    B. False

11. A _____ is something that is definitely true

    A. Opinion

    B. Report

    C. Fact

12. An _____ is something that is may not be true

    A. Opinion

    B. Report

    C. Fact

13. Objective information is based on what you

    A. See

    B. Hear

    C. Touch or smell

    D. All of the above

14. _____ information is something you cannot or did not observe

    A. Objective

    B. Subjective

    C. Rejective

15. Incontinence is

    A. Inability to control moving

    B. Inability to control the bladder or bowels

    C. Inability to control breathing

16. A resident's skin is pale or blue. This is called

    A. Edema

    B. Syncope

    C. Cyanotic

17. Derma means

    A. Head

    B. Neck

    C. Skin

18. The suffix " itis" means

    A. Incontinence

    B. Incision

C. Complication

D. Inflammation

19. _____ is an accident or unexpected event during the course of care

A. Incident

B. Impairment

C. Liability

Match the following

20. Hemiplegia_____	A. medical term for stroke
21. Hemiparesis _____	B. difficulty swallowing
22. Expressive aphasia _____	C. Inability to speak clearly
23. Receptive _____	D. inability to speak clearly
24. Dysphasia ___	E. weakness on one side of the body
25. Cerebrovascular accident (CVA) _____	F. Paralysis on one side the body

SECTION FIVE

1. _____ is term for measures practiced in healthcare facilities to prevent and control the spread of disease

A. Medical asepsis

B. Microbes

C. Infection control

2. A _____ is a living thing or organism that is so small that it can be seen only through a microscope

A. Virus

B. Microorganism

C. Infection

3. What is another name for microorganism

A. Microbe

B. Amoeba

C. Bacteria

4. Infection occur when harmful microorganisms called pathogens invade the body and multiply

True
False
None of the above

5. Which of the following infection is in the blood stream and is spread throughout the body

A. Healthcare-associated infection

B. Localized infection

C. Systemic infection

6. A _____ is confined to a specific location in the body and has local symptoms

A. Healthcare-associated infection

B. Localized infection

C. Systemic infection

7. _____ are infections that patients acquire within healthcare settings that result from treatment for other conditions

A. Healthcare-associated infection

B. Localized infection

C. Systemic infection

8. _____ is the process of removing pathogens or the state of being free of pathogens

A. Medical asepsis

B. Surgical asepsis

C. None of the above

9. What is the name given to the state of being free of all microorganisms not just pathogens

    A. Medical asepsis

    B. Surgical asepsis

    C. None of the above

10. The chain of infection is

    A. Is an uninfected person who could get sick

    B. Is a way of describing how disease is transmitted from one living being to another

    C. None of the above

11. Causative agents include which of the following

    A. Bacteria

    B. Viruses

    C. Fungi and protozoa

    D. All of the above

12. Examples of reservoirs include the

    A. Mouth

    B. Clothes

    C. Lungs, blood and the large intestine

13. The _____ is anybody opening on an infected person that allows pathogens to leave such as the nose, mouth, eyes or a cut in the skin

    A. Portal of entry

    B. Portal of exit

    C. None of the above

14. Which of the following describes how the pathogen travels from one person to the next person

    A. Mode of transmission

    B. Susceptible host

    C. None of the above

15. _____ is the condition that results from inadequate fluid in the body

    A. Infection

    B. Diarrhea

    C. Malnutrition

    D. Dehydration

16. Centers for Disease Control and prevention (CDC) is a governmental agency under the department of health and human services

    True
    False
    None of the above
17. Hand antisepsis refers to

    A. Hand-washing with either plain or antiseptic soap and water and using alcohol-based hand rubs

    B. Washing hands with water and soap or other detergents that contain an antiseptic agent

    C. None of the above

18. A _____ agent destroys or resists pathogen

    A. Microbes

    B. Microbial

    C. Antimicrobial

19. Personal protective equipment includes

    A. Gloves, gown

B. Masks, goggles and face shields

C. All of the above

20. _____ is a process that kills pathogens but not all microorganisms

A. Disinfection

B. Sterilization

C. Disposal

21. Which of the following are symptoms of hepatitis

A. Chest pain

B. Trouble breathing

C. Mucus

D. None of the above

22. Tuberculosis usually infects the

A. Brain

B. Lungs

C. Heart

23. MRSA stands for

A. Methicillin-resistant staphylococcus aureus

B. Multidrug-resistant

C. None of the above

24. _____ stands for vancomycin-resistant enterococcus

A. HIV

B. TB

C. VRE

25. Which of the following is a spore forming bacteria which can be a part of the normal flora

    A. Enterococci

    B. Staphylococcus aureus

    C. Clostridium difficile

SECTION SIX

1. Which of the following includes our 5 senses

    A. Sight and hearing

    B. Touch and smell

    C. Taste

    D. All of the above

2. _____ is the loss of ability to move all or part of the body

    A. Fracture

    B. Paralysis

    C. Sprain

3. It is very important to try to prevent accidents before they occur

    A. True

    B. False

4. A fracture is

    A. A broken bone

    B. A bleeding bone

    C. A severed bone

5. What fracture cause the greatest number of deaths and can lead to severe health problems

    A. Shoulder

B. Leg

C. Hip

6. The following factors increases the risk for falls, except.

   A. Poor lighting

   B. Upholstery

   C. Slippery or wet floor

   D. Throw rugs

7. _____ means confusion about person, place or time

   A. orientation

   B. disorientation

   C. identification

8. Never lock a wheel chair before transferring a resident into or out of it

   A. True

   B. False

9. What can be caused by dry heat ?

   A. Burns

   B. Cuts

   C. Scalds

10. Scalds are burns

A. True

B. False

11. _____ can occur when eating, drinking or swallowing medication

   A. Poisoning

   B. Gasping

C. Slippery

D. Choking

12. Residents must be sitting up straight when eating whether in a bed or a chair

A. True

B. False

13. An _____ is an injury that rubs off the surface of the skin

A. Abrasion

B. Cut

C. Scratch

14. _____ means the process of burning

A. Flammable

B. Smoking

C. Combustion

15. Which of the following requires that all hazardous chemicals must have a material safety data sheet ?

A. MRSA

B. HIV

C. OSHA

16. Which of the following are examples of physical restraints

A. Mitt restraints

B. Belt restraints

C. Side rails

D. All of the above

17. _____ is death from a lack of air or oxygen

A. Suffocation

B. Atrophy

C. Syncope

18. Understanding some basic principles of body mechanisms will help keep you and residents safe

A. True

B. False

19. _____ is the way the parts of the body with together whenever you move

A. Posture

B. Center of gravity

C. Body mechanics

20. Always try to catch a falling resident

A. True

B. False

21. Where does the center of gravity in your body point?

A. Where the most weight is concentrated

B. Where the least weight is concentrated

C. Where no weight is concentrated

22. The wider your support the more stable you are

A. True

B. False

23. A _____ moves an object by resting on a base of support

A. Alignment

B. Lever

C. Counter of gravity

24. When you stand your weight is centered in your pelvis

    A. True

    B. False

25. Do not twist while you are moving an object

A. True

B. False

SECTION SEVEN

1. The first thing to do when you recognize a medical emergency is

    A. Turn on the AED

    B. Do nothing

    C. Assess the situation

    D. Start CPR

2. Which of the following means being mentally alert and having awareness of surroundings, sensations and thoughts?

    A. Conscious

    B. Breathing

    C. Unconscious

    D. None of the above

3. Checking a person for injury include all of the following except

    A. Medical alert tags

    B. Applying restraints

    C. Severe bleeding

    D. Changes in consciousness

4. _____ is an emergency care given immediately to an injured person

    A. CPR

    B. Abdominal thrust

    C. BLS

    D. First aid

5. To open the airway you should use the

    A. Head tilt-chin lift

    B. Chin lift head tilt

    C. Both a and b

    D. None of the above

6. When giving CPR the correct rate of chest compressions to breaths are

    A. 15 chest compressions to 1 rescue breaths

    B. 30 chest compressions to 2 rescue breaths

    C. 20 chest compressions to 1 rescue breaths

    D. 35 chest compressions to 2 rescue breaths

7. AED stands for

    A. Automatic external defibrillator

    B. Auto external defibrillator

    C. Automated externally defibrillator

    D. Automated external defibrillator

8. Adequate breathing should be detected no longer than _____ seconds

    A. 15

    B. 5

    C. 10

D. 20

9. How could you tell when someone is choking

    A. He/she would put their hands to their throat and cough

    B. He/she would ask you to hit them on the back

    C. He/she would ask for a glass of water

    D. None of the above

10. The method of attempting to remove an object from the airway of someone who is choking is called_____

    A. Abdominal slaps

    B. Abdominal thrusts

    C. Depressions

    D. Compressions

11. What occurs when organs and tissues in the body do not receive an adequate blood supply?

    A. Choking

    B. Dyspnea

    C. Syncope

    D. Shock

12. Dyspnea means

    A. Difficulty breathing

    B. Difficulty smelling

    C. Painful breathing

    D. Both a and c

13. All of the following are signs and symptoms of MI except

    A. Nausea and vomiting

B. Perspiration

C. Blurred vision

D. Cold and clammy skin

14. What is the medical term used for heart attack?

    A. Myocardial Ischemia

    B. Myocardial infarction (MI)

    C. Myocardium infarction

    D. None of the above

15. What should be done to control bleeding?

    A. With gloves on and clean, thick sterile pad press down hard directly on the bleeding wound until help arrive

    B. Press down hard directly on the bleeding wound with bare hands until help arrive

    C. Maintain normal body temperature

    D. All of the above

16. Which of the following is used to treat accidental poisoning

    A. Epsom salts

    B. Ipecac syrup

    C. Activated charcoal

    D. All of the above

17. _____ degree burns involves all three layers of the skin

    A. First degree

    B. Second degree

    C. Third degree

    D. Total degree

18. What is the medical term for fainting

A. BLS

B. Syncope

C. Myocardial ischemia

D. Myocardial infarction

19. Insulin reaction is also called

A. Hypoglycemia

B. Hypokalemia

C. Hyperglycemia

D. Hyperkalemia

20. _____ is caused by having too little insulin

A. Hypoglycemia

B. Hyperkalemia

C. Diabetic ketoacidosis (DKA)/hyperglycemia

D. None of the above

21. Which of the following is not a true statement about seizures

A. Do not leave a person alone during a seizure

B. Help the person get up slowly while having a seizure

C. Do not give liquid or food

D. Do not try to restrain the person

22. _____ is a warning sign of a CVA

A. Myocardial ischemia

B. Syncope

C. Emesis

D. Epilepsy

23. Transient ischemic attack (TIA) is also known as

    A. Mini stroke

    B. Semi stroke

    C. Bi-lateral stroke

    D. Tri lateral stroke

24. The act of ejecting stomach contents through the mouth is

    A. Sputum

    B. Mucus

    C. Vomiting or emesis

    D. None of the above

25. Disasters can include

    A. Fire, flood

    B. Earthquake, hurricane

    C. Severe weather

    D. All of the above

SECTION EIGHT

1. Which of the following is the correct order of Maslow's hierarchy of needs

    A. Self-esteem, belongingness, self-actualization

    B. Safety, physical needs, love and belongingness, security

    C. Self-actualization, self-esteem, belongingness and security

    D. Physical need, safety and security, love and belongingness, self-esteem and self-actualization

2. Considering a whole system such as a whole person rather than dividing the system up into parts

A. Holistic

B. Mental

C. Independence

D. None of the above

3. Which of the following is not a basic human physical need

    A. Safety

    B. Food and water

    C. Getting an ipad

    D. Comfort

4. A loss of independence can cause which of the following

    A. Depression

    B. Poor self- image

    C. Feelings of being useless

    D. All of the above

5. _____ means to touch or rub sexual organs in order to give oneself or another person sexual pleasure

    A. Mensuration

    B. Masturbation

    C. Menstruation

    D. Menopause

6. A person who has a desire for persons of the same sex is called a

    A. Transsexual

    B. Bisexual

    C. Heterosexual

D. Gay

7. A woman whose sexual orientation is to women

   A. Lesbian

   B. Gay

   C. Transsexual

   D. Bisexual

8. Spirituality means

   A. Relating to the spirit or soul

   B. Relating to the mind

   C. Relating to the way we conduct our selves

   D. None of the above

Fill in the blank
Atheists   Buddhism   Christianity   Islam   Judaism   Islam
9. Believe that life is filled with suffering that caused by desire _____

10. Believe Jesus Christ was the son of God and that he died so their sins would be forgiven _____

11. Believe in reincarnation, karma and do not eat beef _____

12. Pray five times a day facing Mecca, the holy city for their religion _____

13. People who claim that there is no God _____

14. Do not do work from Friday sundown to Saturday sundown _____

15. Fasting means

    A. Eating vegan food

    B. Eating soul food

    C. Not eating food or eating very little food

D. None of the above

16. _____ do not eat any animals or animal products such as eggs or dairy products

A. Vegetarian

B. Vegans

C. Ovo vegetarians

D. Lacto vegetarians

17. A highly contagious viral disease that strikes nearly all children is

A. Leukemia

B. SIDS

C. Ageism

D. Chicken pox

18. _____ is a maltreatment include not providing adequate food, clothing or support

A. Child neglect

B. Trauma

C. Premature

D. Disability

19. School-age children age from

A. 12 to 18

B. 3 to 6

C. 6 to 12

D. 18 to 40

20. _____ is a form of cancer

A. Chicken pox

B. Bulimia

C. Leukemia

D. SIDS

21. What is the study of health, wellness and disease later in life

A. Gerontology

B. Geriatrics

C. Ageism

D. Cognitive

22. The study of the aging process in people from mid-life through old age is called

A. Scientology

B. Geriatrics

C. Zoology

D. Gerontology

23. Prejudice towards stereotyping of against older persons or the elderly is called

A. Ageism

B. Anorexia

C. Old age

D. Gigantism

24. _____ refer to disabilities that are at birth or emerge during child-hood

A. Developmental disabilities

B. Down syndrome

C. Spina bifida

D. Cerebral palsy

25. Spina bifida literally means

A. Crack spine

B. Rip spine

C. Split spine

D. Age spine

SECTION NINE

1. What is the name for the condition in which all of the body's systems are working at their best

   A. Homeostasis

   B. Hormones

   C. Glands

   D. Digestion

2. The body is divided into _____ systems

   A. 7

   B. 9

   C. 10

   D. 11

3. Body systems are made up of

   A. Cells

   B. Glands

   C. Tissues

   D. Organs

4. What are the building block of our bodies

   A. Organs

   B. Cells

C. Tissues

D. Glands

5. Posterior or dorsal means

   A. Away from the body

   B. The back of the body or body part

   C. The front of the body or body part

   D. Closer to the torso

6. The largest organ and system in the body is the

   A. Skin

   B. Endocrine

   C. Reproductive

   D. Musculoskeletal

7. Normal changes of aging include which of the following

   A. Skin is less elastic

   B. Nails are harder and more brittle

   C. Hair thins and may turn gray

   D. All of the above

8. Which of the following is not a part of the skin

   A. Epidermis

   B. Dermis

   C. Epicardium

   D. Subcutaneous

9. How many bones are there in the human body?

   A. 206

B. 210

C. 220

D. 212

10. The point at where two bones meet is called a

    A. Tissue

    B. Contract

    C. Glands

    D. Joint

11. _____ provide movement of body parts to maintain posture and to produce heat

    A. Joint

    B. Muscles

    C. Cells

    D. Organs

12. Which of the following is not included in normal changes of aging

    A. Bone loss density

    B. Muscles weaken and lose tone

    C. Height is gradually lost

    D. Grow 6 inches taller

13. Which one of the following is the two main parts of the nervous system

    A. Central nervous system (CNS)

    B. Peripheral nervous system

    C. A and B

    D. None of the above

14. The three main sections of the brain are

A. Cerebrum

B. Brainstem

C. Cerebellum

D. All of the above

15. The outer part of the eye is called

A. Sclera

B. Retina

C. Iris

D. Cornea

16. Ear wax and hair in the ear protect the ear from

A. Light

B. Foreign objects

C. Water

D. None of the above

17. The heart is an

A. Bone

B. Organ

C. Muscle

D. Artery

18. The contracting phase of the heart is the

A. Expiration

B. Diastole

C. Systole

D. Inspiration

19. The resting phase of the heart is the

    A. Diastole

    B. Respiration

    C. Inspiration

    D. Expiration

20. Normal changes of aging include which of the following

    A. Voice weakens

    B. Lung capacity decreases

    C. Lung strength decreases

    D. All of the above

21. _____ is the process of expelling solid wastes made up of the waste products of food that are not absorbed into cells

    A. Digestion

    B. Ingestion

    C. Absorption

    D. Elimination

22. Fecal/anal incontinence is the

    A. Inability to control the bowels

    B. Inability to control urine

    C. Inability to control drooling

    D. Inability to control bleeding

23. The reproductive system allows human beings to _____

    A. Multiply

    B. Separate

C. Reproduce

D. None of the above

24. _____ protects against a particular disease that is invading the body at a given time

    A. Acquired immunity

    B. Specific immunity

    C. Nonspecific immunity

    D. Invading immunity

25. What is the name of the clear yellowish fluid that carries disease-fighting cells called lymphocytes

    A. Sperm

    B. Lymph

    C. Gonads

    D. None of the above

SECTION TEN

1. _____ means helping residents into positions that will be comfortable and healthy for them

    A. Positioning

    B. Homeostasis

    C. Holistic

2. In the _____ position the resident lies flat on his back

    A. Lateral

    B. Prone

    C. Supine

3. A person in the _____ position is lying on his or her back

A. Prone

B. Lateral

C. Supine

4. A person lying in the _____ position is lying on his or her stomach

A. Prone

B. Sims

C. Fowlers

5. A person lying in the _____ position is partially reclined

A. Prone

B. Sims

C. Fowlers

6. A draw sheet is an extra sheet placed on top of the bottom sheet

A. True

B. False

7. _____ is rubbing or friction that results from the skin moving one way and the bone underneath it remaining fixed or moving in the opposite direction

A. Shearing

B. Bearing

C. Shaving

8. Moving a resident as a unit, without disturbing alignment of the body is

A. Block rolling

B. Wood rolling

C. Log rolling

9. To _____means to sit up with the feet over the side of the bed for a moment to regain balance

A. Swing

B. Dangle

C. Shake

10. The science of designing equipment and work tasks to suit the workers abilities

A. Transfer board

B. Ergonomics

C. Gait belt

11. A _____ is a safety device used to transfer residents who are weak, unsteady or uncoordinated

A. Transfer belt

B. Gait belt

C. Safety belt

12. Where should the gait belt be placed?

A. Around both legs of the resident

B. Around the waist of resident over clothing

C. On the wheel chair

13. What is the name of the equipment that can help transfer residents?

A. Back belt

B. holding belt

C. Gait belt

14. A stretcher is another word for

A. Cane

B. Gurney

C. Crutch

15. Which of the following equipment prevents wear and tear on your body

A. Stretcher

B. Mechanical or hydraulic lift

C. Sling

16. Which of the following statements are not true about a mechanical lift?

    A. You and the resident would not get hurt if you use the lift improperly

    B. You must be trained on the specific lift you will be using

    C. Lifts help prevent injury to you and the resident

17. Which of the following statements are true about transferring a resident onto and off a toilet

    A. Position wheelchair at a right angle to toilet

    B. Ask resident to push against the arm rests of the wheelchair and stand

    C. All of the above

18. What is another word for walking?

    A. Ambulation

    B. Pacing

    C. Moving

19. A resident who is ambulatory is

    A. One who can move in bed

    B. One who can get out of bed and walk

    C. None of the above

20. The purpose of a cane is to

    A. Help with balance

    B. Help visually impaired resident

    C. None of the above

21. The _____ cane is a straight cane with a curved handle at the top

    A. C cane

    B. Quad cane

    C. Functional grip cane

22. This type of cane has a grip handle rather than a curved handle

    A. C cane

    B. Quad cane

    C. Functional grip cane

23. Which cane is designed to bear more weight than the other canes

    A. C cane

    B. Quad cane

    C. Functional grip cane

24. What equipment can be used when the resident can bear some weight on the legs

    A. Walker

    B. Cane

    C. Crutches

25. Residents who can bear no weight or limited weight on the leg use

    A. Walker

    B. Cane

    C. Crutches

SECTION ELEVEN

Fill in the blanks

Wants, them   time, condition   consciousness confused   introduce position

Friendly formal resident arrives bed tidy admission kit welcome, wanted tour valuables

1. Prepare the room before the resident _____

2. Make sure the _____ is made and the room is _____

3. A _____ _____ is usually in the patient room before he/she is admitted

4. When a new resident arrives at the facility note the _____ and _____

5. Observe the new resident for level of _____ and if he/she seems _____

6. _____ yourself and state your _____

7. Smile and be _____

8. Always call the person by his/her _____ name until they tell you what they want to be call

9. Never rush the new _____

10. Make sure the new resident feel _____ and _____

11. Offer to take the resident on a _____

12. Ask the new resident if he/she brought any _____

13. Place personal items where the resident _____ _____

True and False
14. Providing fresh water is something you should do every time you leave a resident's room

15. Report any changes in resident's weight to the nurse

16. Residents do not have the right to receive advance notice of any room or roommate change

17. Sphygmomanometer is used to measure blood pressure

18. Alcohol wipes cannot be used for infection and minor wound care

19. Otoscope is an instrument used to examine the eye

20. The dorsal recumbent position is used to examine the chest, breasts and abdomen

21. Lithotomy position is used to examine the rectum

22. To determine height on a standing scale gently lower the measuring rod until it rests flat on the resident's head

23. Admission kit will contain a urine specimen cup, personal care items, drinking glass, tooth paste and soap

24. Resident should not be told of their rights until after admission

25. The room should be prepare when the new resident arrives

SECTION TWELVE

True and false

1. Illness and disability cause great stress

2. Common noises in facilities can upset and irritate residents

3. Caffeinated drinks such as coffee or some teas do not prevent sleep, fatigue and irritability

4. A resident room is not his/her home and should not be treated with respect

5. Providing a clean, safe and orderly environment is an essential part of your job

6. Normally Beds are kept at their highest horizontal position

7. The water pitcher and cup are kept in the bedside stand drawer

8. It is important to always place the call light within the resident's reach

9. Curtains and screens block sounds from the other rooms

10. You do not have to wear gloves when rinsing bedpans and urinals

11. Sleep is a natural period of rest for the mind and body

12. The circadian rhythm is 24 hour day night cycle

13. Insomnia is the lack of ability to fall asleep or stay asleep

14. Sheets that are damp, wrinkled or bunched up under a resident is not uncomfortable

15. Hold soiled linen close to your body and place it in the proper container immediately

16. An occupied bed is a bed made while the resident is not in it

17. It is easier to make a bed when the resident is in it

18. Hospital corners help keep the flat sheet smooth under the resident

19. A close bed is a bed completely made with the bedspread and blankets in place

20. A surgical bed is made to accept residents who are returning to bed on stretchers or gurney

21. Good lighting is not important to residents

22. Always knock and wait to receive permission before entering

23. If resident seem sad, anxious, or fearful just ignore them

24. You do not have to keep a resident room neat and clean

25. An emesis basin is a kidney-shaped basin often used when giving mouth care

SECTION THIRTEEN

1. _____ is the term used to describe practices to keep our bodies clean and healthy

    A. Hygiene

    B. Grooming

    C. ADL

    D. None of the above

2. What is refered to as practices like caring for fingernails and hair

    A. Hygiene

    B. Grooming

    C. ADL

    D. None of the above

3. Which of the following is not included in a.m. care

    A. Offering a bedpan

B. Giving a back rub

C. Helping the resident to wash face and hands

D. Assisting with mouth care before breakfast

4. _____ are areas of the body that bear much of its weight

   A. Pressure sores

   B. Bony prominences

   C. Pressure points

   D. None of the above

5. The areas of the body where the bone lies close to the skin is

   A. Pressure sore

   B. Pressure points

   C. Hygiene

   D. Bony prominences

6. A pressure sore is also called a

   A. Decubitus ulcer

   B. Pressure points

   C. Broken skin

   D. None of the above

7. How many stages of pressure sores exists?

   A. 2

   B. 4

   C. 3

   D. 5

8. In what stage is the full skin loss with major destruction

A. Stage 1

B. Stage 2

C. Stage 4

D. Stage 3

9. In what stage is the skin intact but there is redness that is not relieved within 15 to 30 minutes?

A. Stage 4

B. Stage 2

C. Stage 3

D. Stage 1

10. A _____ skin or _____ skin may be placed under the resident to absorb moisture

A. Goat, pig

B. Cow, dog

C. Sheep, chamois

D. None of the above

11. _____ heel protectors help keep feet properly aligned and prevent pressure sores

A. Stuffed

B. Padded

C. Packed

D. Shield

12. There are many types of ointments, creams and lotions that are used to treat, soften and protect the skin

A. True

B. False

C. Maybe

D. None of the above

13. _____ is a weakness of muscles in the feet and ankles that causes difficulty with the ability to flex the ankles and walk normally

   A. Foot pop

   B. Foot roll

   C. Foot curl

   D. Foot drop

14. What help prevent foot drop?

   A. Footboards

   B. Foot stools

   C. Foot roll

   D. Foot curls

15. Hand rolls does not keep fingers from curling too tightly

   A. True

   B. False

16. A _____ is a device such as a splint or brace that helps support and align a limb and improve its function

   A. Splint device

   B. Brace device

   C. Orthotic device

   D. Pillow device

17. The perineum is the

   A. Vocal and skin area

   B. Mucus and genital area

C. Genital and back area

D. Genital and anal area

18. A _____ is a substance added to another substance changing its effect

A. Additive

B. Subtractive

C. Partial

D. None of the above

19. Common sites for pressure sores are

A. Thigh

B. Shoulder

C. Chest, nose and hands

D. None of the above

20. The _____ is the area from the pubis to the upper thighs

A. Buttock

B. Groin

C. Abdomen

D. Perineal

21. A _____ is a sturdy chair designed to be placed in a bathtub or shower

A. Geri chair

B. Wheel chair

C. Shower chair

D. None of the above

22. Pediculosis is an

A. Infestation of mice

B. Infestation of pest

C. Infestation of bugs

D. Infestation of lice

23. _____ is an excessive shedding of dead skin cells from the scalp

A. Scab

B. Dandruff

C. Scratch

D. Crack

24. The medical term for bad breath is

A. Edentulous

B. Aspiration

C. Halitosis

D. Pediculosis

25. Edentulous means

A. Having no teeth

B. Having no sweat

C. Having no pain

D. Having bad breath

SECTION FOURTEEN

1. Which of the following is the normal temperature range for the oral method

A. 96.6 - 98.6 degrees F

B. 97.9 - 100.6 degrees F

C. 97.6 - 99.6 degrees F

D. 95.6 - 98.9 degrees F

2. Which of the following is the normal temperature range for the rectal method

    A. 98.6 - 100.6 degrees F

    B. 96.7 - 98.6 degrees F

    C. 95.6 – 98.9 degrees F

    D. 98.6 – 99.9 degrees F

3. Which of the following is another word for mouth

    A. Axillary

    B. Rectal

    C. Tympanic

    D. Oral

4. Which of the following is another word for ear

    A. Axillary

    B. Rectal

    C. Tympanic

    D. Oral

5. Oral thermometers are usually _____ in color

    A. Yellow

    B. Green or blue

    C. Black

    D. Lavender

6. Rectal thermometers are usually _____ in color

    A. Yellow

    B. Green

C. Blue

D. Red

7. Which temperature is considered to be the most accurate?

   A. Rectal

   B. Oral

   C. Tympanic

   D. Axillary

8. Which temperature is considered to be the least accurate?

   A. Oral

   B. Tympanic

   C. Axillary

   D. Rectal

9. Why are mercury free thermometers safer than the mercury thermometers?

   A. They are more expensive than mercury thermometers

   B. They do not contain dangerous substance like mercury

   C. They are easier to read than mercury thermometers

   D. They are easier to hold

10. Where is the most common site for monitoring the pulse located

    A. In between the elbow and the shoulder

    B. In between the thigh and the leg

    C. On the feet

    D. On the inside of the wrist

11. Where is the brachial pulse located

    A. In between the elbow and the shoulder

B. On the side of the neck

C. On the feet

D. On the left side of the chest

12. Which of the following is not a common pulse site?

A. Radial

B. Apical

C. Femoral

D. All of the above

13. A _____ is an instrument designed to listen to sounds within the body

A. Sphygmomanometer

B. Stethoscope

C. Pen

D. Thermometer

14. What is the process of breathing air into the lungs?

A. Perspiration

B. Dyspnea

C. Respiration

D. Expiring

15. Count the heart beat for _____ full minute to measure apical pulse

A. 1

B. 3

C. 2

D. 4

16. The normal respiration rate for adults ranges from

A. 40 to 60

B. 12 to 16

C. 15 to 30

D. 12 to 20

17. Infants normally breath at a rate of _____ to _____ cycles per minute

A. 24 to 30

B. 15 to 35

C. 30 to 40

D. 12 to 16

True and false

18. Heat relieves pain and muscular tension

19. Hot application can stop bleeding

20. Ice packs is considered to be a dry applicator

21. Disposable heat compresses are used more than once and then discarded

22. Sitz baths clean perineal wounds and reduce inflammation and pain

23. Sterile dressing do not cover open or drain wounds

24. IV stands for intravenous or into a vein

25. A nasal cannula is a piece of metal tubing that fits around the face

SECTION FIFTEEN

1. _____ is how the body uses food to maintain health

A. Carbohydrates

B. Nutrition

C. Fats

D. Protein

2. What is something found in food that provides energy, promote good health and helps regulate metabolism

    A. Oil

    B. Fat

    C. Vegetables

    D. Nutrient

3. _____promotes growth

    A. Protein

    B. Grains

    C. Minerals

    D. Fruits

4. Carbohydrates are basically needed for _____

    A. growth

    B. strength

    C. None of the above

5. Fats help the body store _____

    A. Vegetables

    B. Fruits

    C. Energy

    D. Milk

6. Vitamins _____,_____, _____ and _____ are fat-soluble vitamins

    A. A, D, E and K

B. B, C and D

C. K, B, and E

D. None of the above

7. Which of the following is not an example of a mineral

A. Zinc, iron

B. Calcium

C. Magnesium

D. Vitamin b

8. One- half to two-thirds of our body weight is

A. Fat

B. Water

C. Food

D. Blood

9. Calcium is used for building _____ and _____

A. Hair and skin

B. Fingers and toes

C. Bones and teeth

D. Nose and mouth

10. _____ are the major source of monounsaturated fats (MUFA)

A. Oils

B. Milk

C. Beans

D. Meat

True or false

11. Physical activity and nutrition work together for better health

12. Many elderly people take a variety of medications which can affect the way food smells and tastes

13. Thickened liquid include water and juice

14. Nasogastric tube are inserted in through the stomach

15. Nursing assistants are responsible for inserting and discontinuing tubes

16. Food likes and dislikes are influenced by what you eat as a child

17. The dietary department also makes diet cards

Match the following

18. Low sodium diet _____   A. Nothing by mouth

19. Dysphagia _____   B. Restricted protein

20. Vegetarians _____   C. clear juices, broth, gelatin and popsicles

21. High-potassium diets ___   D. Helps with constipation

22. NPO _____   E. Do not eat fish or poultry

23. Low-protein diet _____   F. No salt added

24. Liquid diet _____   G. Get food high in potassium (Banana, grapefruit)

25. High-residue diet _____ H. Difficulty swallowing

SECTION SIXTEEN

1. Urination is also known as

   A. Number 1

   B. Defaecation

   C. Micturition or voiding

   D. None of the above

2. Urine is made up of

    A. Fruits and vegetables

    B. Water and dye

    C. Mucus and water

    D. Water and waste products

3. Adults should produce about _____ to _____ mL of urine per day

    A. 2000 to 4000

    B. 1200 to 1500

    C. 400 to 600

    D. 60 to 100

4. Urine is normally _____ to _____ in color

    A. Pale yellow to amber

    B. Pale pink to red

    C. Pale yellow to orange

    D. Green to blue

5. A healthy person needs to take in from _____ of fluid each day

    A. 30 to 60 ounces

    B. 20 to 40 ounces

    C. 50 to 70 ounces

    D. 64 to 96 ounces

6. _____ is a bedpan that is flatter than the regular bedpan

    A. Woven pan

    B. Twisted pan

    C. Fracture pan

D. Standard pan

7. Urinary tract infection (UTI) causes

    A. Inflammation of the kidney and nephron

    B. Inflammation of the bladder and ureters

    C. Inflammation of the perineal area

    D. None of the above

8. Another name for kidney stones is

    A. Calculi

    B. Calculus

    C. Catheter

    D. Cystitis

9. Which of the following is not a symptom of calculi?

    A. Groin pain

    B. Chills, fever

    C. Sore throat

    D. Flank or back pain

10. Inflammation of the kidneys is

    A. Cystitis

    B. Nephritis

    C. Edema

    D. None of the above

11. _____ is a condition in which a blockage of arteries in the kidneys causes high blood pressure

    A. Ranovascular hypertension

B. Rinovascular hypertension

C. Renovascular hypotension

D. Renovascular hypertension

True OR False

12. Excessive salt in the diet can also cause damage to the kidney

13. A catheter is a thick tube inserted in the body

14. Nursing assistant insert, remove and irrigate catheter

15. Straight catheter remains inside the body

16. Indwelling catheter is removed immediately after urine is drained

17. Kidney dialysis is an artificial means of removing the body's waste products

18. A specimen is a sample that is used for analysis in order to try make a diagnosis

19. A clean catch specimen is also called mid-stream because the first and last is not included

20. The pH scale ranges from 0 to 14

21. Normal pH of urine range from 8.4 – 9.0

22. Kidney stones are produced when the body burns fat for fuel

23. Illness and diseases can cause blood to appear in the urine

24. Always show anger and frustration toward resident who are incontinent

25. Never report changes in skin color

SECTION SEVENTEEN

True and false

1. Defecation or bowel elimination is the passing of feces from the large intestine out of the body through the anus

2. Feces is also called stool or bowel movement

3. Stool is normally black, hard and formed in a tubular shape

4. Certain food can change the color of stool

5. Liquid stool should be reported to the nurse

6. As a person ages peristalsis increase

7. Raw fruits and vegetables are high in fiber which helps with bowel movement

8. Constipation is the ability to eliminate urine

Fill in the blank

BRAT   Colitis   Malabsorption   Harris flush   Weakening   Peptic Ulcers
120 ml   Blood   Worms and amoebas   Occult   Colon cancer
Enema   Fecal impaction   Hemorrhoids   Diarrhea   Flatus or gas   lactose intolerance

9. A specific amount of water with or without an additive that is introduced into the colon to eliminate stool is _____

10. A _____ _____ is a hard stool that is stuck in the rectum and cannot be expelled

11. _____ are enlarged veins in the rectum that may also be visible outside the anus

12. Frequent elimination of liquid or semi-liquid feces is called _____

13. Flatulence is also called _____ or _____

14. The inability to digest lactose a type of sugar found in milk and other dairy products is called _____

15. A diet of bananas, rice, applies and tea/ toast is also called _____ diet

16. Irritable bowel movement syndrome which is a chronic form of stomach upset that gets worse from stress is _____

17. _____ means that the body cannot absorb or digest a particular nutrient properly

18. A return-flow enema also called a _____ may be ordered to expel the flatus

19. Heartburn is the result of a _____ of the sphincter muscle which joins the esophagus and the stomach

20. _____ are raw sores in the stomach or the small intestine

21. Colorectal cancer also known as _____ is cancer of the gastrointestinal tact

22. A commercially-prepared enema usually has _____ solution and may have additives

23. Stool specimens are collected so that the stool can be tested for _____

24. _____ and _____ can be detected with an ova and parasites test

25. _____ means something that is hidden or difficult to see or observe

SECTION EIGHTEEN

Fill in the blank

Vaginitis   Sarcoptes scabiei   hyperthyroidism   myocardial infarction   angina pectoris
Atherosclerosis   glaucoma   safe   spinal cord   impairments   circulation   Parkinson
Right   CVA   complimentary medicine   amputation   muscular dystrophy (MD)
Closed   women   autoimmune illness   ringworm   itching   inflammation   wound
shingles

1. Scabies is a skin condition caused by a tiny mite called _____

2. _____ is also called herpes zoster

3. A _____ is a type of injury to the skin

4. Dermatitis is a general term that refers to an _____ or swelling of the skin

5. Early signs of stasis dermatitis include rash, a scaly red area and _____

6. _____ is a fungal infection that causes red, ring-like patches to appear on the upper body, hands and feet

7. Arthritis may be the result of aging, injury or an _____

8. Osteoporosis is more common in _____ after menopause

9. A _____ fracture is a broken bone that does not break the skin

10. _____ refers to several progressive diseases that cause a variety of physical disabilities due to muscle weakness

11. What is the removal of some or all of a body part, usually a foot, hand arm or leg

12. Treatment that are used in addition to the conventional treatments prescribed by a doctor is refer to as _____

13. _____ or stroke is caused when the blood supply to the brain is cut off suddenly by a clot or a ruptured blood vessel

14. Weaknesses on the _____ side show that the left side of the brain was affected

15. A person with _____ disease may have a mask-like facial expression

16. Range of motion exercises help prevent contractures, strengthen muscles and increase _____

17. Multiple sclerosis is an unpredictable disease that causes varying symptoms and _____

18. People with _____ injury may have paraplegia or loss of function of lower body and legs

19. During a seizure the main goal of the caregiver is to make sure that the resident is _____

20. _____ is a disease that causes the pressure in the eye to increase

21. Hypertension is caused by _____ or hardening and narrowing of the blood vessels

22. The medical term for chest pain is _____

23. The medical term for heart attack is _____

24. When the thyroid produces too much thyroid hormone the cells burn too much food this is called _____

25. _____ is an infection of the vagina

SECTION NINETEEN
(Match to the correct answer)

1. Cognition ___ A. a progressive degenerative and irreversible disease

2. Confusion ___ B. the time of signs and symptoms

3. Delirium ___   C. disease or condition cannot be cured

4. Dementia ___ D. disease gets worse

5. Progressive __ E. disease is advance

6. Degenerative __F. ability to think logically and quickly

7. Onset __   G. State of severe confusion

8. Irreversible___ H. serious loss of mental abilities

9. Alzheimer's disease ___ I. inability to think clearly

10. In this stage of Alzheimer's the resident would be disoriented to time

    A. Stage I

    B. Stage III

    C. Stage III

    D. Stage IV

11. Which of the following is included in stage II Alzheimer's

    A. Temper tantrums

    B. Incontinence

    C. Inability to read, write or do math

    D. All of the above

12. Which of the following Is not included in Stage III Alzheimer's

    A. Difficulty swallowing

    B. Mood swings

    C. Inability to recognize family or self

    D. Increased sleep disturbances

13. People with Alzheimer's disease will not show all the symptoms at the same time

    A. True

B. False

C. None of the above

D. C only

14. When residents say the same words, phrases or questions or over and over, this is called _____

   A. Reservation

   B. Preservation

   C. Presumption

   D. Repetition

15. Which one of the following words means a way to change an action or development?

   A. Determination

   B. Intervention

   C. Reservation

   D. Prevention

16. A resident who is excited, restless or troubled is said to be_____

   A. Triggers

   B. Sun downing

   C. Agitated

   D. None of the above

17. When a person gets restless and agitated in the late afternoon, evening or night it is called

   A. Triggers

   B. Sun downing

   C. Agitated

   D. None of the above

18. When a person with Alzheimer's disease overreacts to something in an unreasonable way it is called a
A. Sun setting
B. sun downing
C. violent behavior
D. Catastrophic reaction

19. A resident attacks, hits or threatens someone is _____
A. disruptive
B. violent
C. alzhermic
D. dementic

20. Walking back and forth in the same area is called.
A. Pacing
B. wandering
C. Sun downing
D. none of the above

21. A resident who sees things that are not there is having_____.
A. Hallucinations
B. depression
C. delusions
D. none of the above

22. A resident who believes things in a physical disease he has that is not there is suffering from_____
A. hallucinations
B. depression
C. Hypochondriac delusion
D. none of the above

23. _____ is taking things that belong to someone else
A. sun downing
B. catastrophic reaction
C. hoarding
D. pillaging

24. Collecting and putting things away in a guarded way is known as
A. pillaging
B. validating
C. hoarding
D. all of the above

25. Validating means
A. taking things of value
B. touching others
C. putting a stamp on everything
D. giving value to or approving

SECTION TWENTY

MATCH

1. Mental health _____   A. Repeated use of legal or illegal drugs

2. Mental illness _____   B. A method of treating mental illness

3. Fallacy _____   C. Form of disease that centers mainly on hallucinations and
   delusions

4. Denial _____   D. Lack of interest in activities

5. Projection _____   E. Anxiety caused by a traumatic experience

6. Displacement _____   F. Behavior a person uses to cope with anxiety

7. Rationalization _____   G. Causes a person to swing from deep depression to extreme
   activity

8. Repression _____   H. A person is terrified for no known reason

9. Regression _____   I. My cause a person to lose interest in everything

10. Anxiety _____   J. A brain disorder that affects a person's ability to think

11. Phobias _____   K. Intense form of anxiety

12. Claustrophobia _____   L. The fear of being in confined space

13. Panic disorder _____   M. Uneasiness or fear

14. Obsessive compulsive ___ N. Going back to an old immature behavior

15. Post-traumatic stress ____ O. Not remembering sexual abuse

16. Apathy _____   P. Everybody does it

17. Schizophrenia _____   Q. Transferring a strong negative feeling to a safer situation

18. Major depression ___   R. My teacher hates me

19. Manic depression ___   S. Completely rejecting the thought or feeling

20. Paranoid schizophrenia _____ T. False belief

21. Psychotherapy _____   U. A disease

22. Substance abuse _____ V. Normal functioning of emotional and intellectual abilities

23. Social interaction can promote mental and physical health

   A. True

   B. False

   C. None of the above

24. Common symptoms of anxiety include which of the following

   A. Muscle aches

   B. Dry mouth

   C. Shakiness

   D. All of the above

25. Which of the following is not a common symptom of schizophrenia

   A. Lack of energy

   B. Irritability

   C. Little or no interest in surroundings

SECTION TWENTY ONE
MATCH

1. Rehabilitation _____   A. Use when resident cannot move on their own

2. Trapeze _____   B. Performed by resident himself

3. Prosthesis _____   C. Moving body part away from the midline of the body

4. ROM _____   D. moving body part towards the midline of the body

5. PROM _____   E. Bending backward

6. AROM _____   F. Device that replaces a body part

7. AAROM _____   G. Turning a joint

8. Abduction _____   H. Triangular piece of equipment that hangs over the head of the bed

9. Adduction _____   I. Straightening a body part

10. Dorsiflexion _____   J. Bending a body part

11. Rotation _____   K. Turning upward

12. Extension _____   L. Care that is managed by professionals to help restore a person

13. Flexion _____   M. Turning downward

14. Pronation _____   N. Done by the resident with some assistance

15. Supination _____   O. Exercise that puts a joint through its full arc of motion

Fill in the blank

Incentive spirometer   lungs   increase circulation   belts, cuffs or suction   trapeze   plate guard

Lower   high blood pressure   physical and mental health   rehabilitation

16. _____ and restorative care is one of the great joy of working as a care giver

17. Exercise is important for improving and maintaining _____ and _____ health

18. Exercising with _____ can be risky

19. Cool-down exercises are done to slowly _____ the heart rate

20. _____ prevent food from being pushed off the plate and make it easier to scoop food onto utensils

21. People in bed can grasp a _____ with their hands which enables them to lift themselves

22. Most artificial limbs are attached by _____

23. The goal of ROM is to decrease or prevent contractures, improve strength and

_____

24. Deep breathing exercise help expand the _____ clearing them of mucus and preventing infections

25. _____ are used for deep breathing exercises

SECTION TWENTY TWO

True and false

1. Sub-acute care is a kind of specialized care that falls between acute care and long term care

2. Dialysis cleanses the body of waste that the kidneys cannot remove due to chronic kidney failure

3. Anesthesia medication do not help pain

4. Before surgery there will be an order for the patient to eat as much as they want

5. A person who is having surgery will require preoperative physical preparation as well

6. NPO means you can have water but no food

7. Postoperative care begins right after surgery

8. A pulse oximeter is an invasive device that uses a light to determine the amount of oxygen in the blood

9. Normal blood oxygen level usually measures between 95% and 100%

10. Telemetry is used to measure the heart rhythm and rate on a continuous basis

11. An artificial airway is any plastic, metal or rubber device inserted into the respiratory tract to maintain or promote breathing

12. There is only one type of artificial airway

13. A sensor is a clip on a person's finger, earlobe, or toe

Fill in the blank

Doctor   nostrils flaring   membrane, covers, protects   constipation   compassionate
pleural cavity chest tube   mucus, secretions   sedative   larynx   mechanical ventilation
tracheostomy

14. One type of artificial airway is a _____

15. _____ is using a machine to assist with or replace breathing when a person is unable to do this on their own

16. The vocal cord is also called the _____

17. A _____ is an agent or drug that helps calm and soothe a person and may cause sleep

18. Suctioning removes _____ and _____ from the lungs

19. _____ are hollow drainage tubes that are inserted into the chest during a sterile procedure

20. The _____ is the space between the layers of the pleura

21. Patients often have many worries before surgery but a _____ response by staff may help alleviate concerns

22. Complications of surgery can also include urinary retention or infections, _____, blood pressure variance and blood clots

23. The pleura is the thin _____ that _____ and _____ the lungs

24. Signs of respiratory distress include _____

25. A _____ normally inserts test tubes

SECTION TWENTY THREE

1. A _____ is a disease or condition that will eventually cause death

   A. Stroke

   B. Denial

C. Terminal illness

D. None of the above

2. Who researched and wrote about the grief process?

   A. Elizabeth kubler-Ross

   B. Abraham Maslow

   C. Erik Erikson

   D. Rick Dickson

3. Which of the following includes the five stages of death and dying?

   A. Denial, shock, anger, guilt, depression

   B. Denial, anger, bargaining, depression, acceptance

   C. Anger, depression, regret, loneliness, pain

   D. Pain, hunger, thirst, guilt, fear

4. Slow irregular respirations or rapid shallow respirations are called___

   A. Cheryl-stokes

   B. Cherry-stokes

   C. Chin-stokes

   D. Cheyne-stokes

5. When the muscles in the body become stiff and rigid this is called

   A. Rigor mortis

   B. Reggae mortis

   C. Roger mortis

   D. Rogain mortis

6. _____ is care of the body after death

   A. Premortem care

B. Palliative care

C. Personal care

D. Postmortem care

7. Rigor mortis is a _____ for stiffness of death

A. Greek word

B. Latin word

C. French word

D. German word

8. Which of the following is the removal of organs and tissues for the purpose of transplanting into someone who needs them

A. Organic donation

B. Oregon donation

C. Organ donation

D. Oregano donation

9. PCA means_____

A. Patient-controlled analgesia

B. Patient-care analysis

C. Patient-comfort analysis

D. None of the above

Match the following

10. Denial _____ A. May be surprise of the death of our love ones

11. Anger _____ B. May regret things we said or did not say

12. Bargaining ___ C. We may cry or feel emotionally unstable

13. Depression ___ D. Missing someone who has died

14. Acceptance ___ E. The practices we grow up with

15. Shock _____   F. Allow people to choose what medical care they want or do not want

16. Regret _____   G. Plan for their last days or ceremony

17. Sadness _____   H. Denying or refusing to believe we are grieving

18. Loneliness _____ I. Cry or withdraw

19. Cultural background _____ J. make promises to God

20. Advance directive _____ K. We may be angry with ourselves or God

True and false

21. A person who is dying may become depressed and withdrawn

22. The goal of hospice are comfort and dignity of the resident

23. Being a good listener can be a great help to a dying resident and his/her family

24. A DNR tells medical professionals to perform CPR

25. A dying resident's room should be softly lit without glare

SECTION TWENTY FOUR

Fill in the blank

Improve   constructive   polite   internet   health   regularly   proud   support
tolerance   stressor   stress   12 hours   OBRA   suggestions   criticism   B, C   job
description   lie   criminal   resume   called   potential   hands-on   lab technicians
direct service

1. Nursing assistants, doctors and nurses all provide _____

2. _____ may conduct tests to help diagnose a condition

3. Chiropractors perform _____ manipulations or adjustments of the spine or other joints

4. To find a job you must first fine _____ employers

5. References are people who can be _____ to recommend you as an employee

6. A _____ is a summary or listing of relevant job experience and education

7. Never _____ on your job application

8. By law employer must perform a _____ background check on all new aides hired

9. A _____ is an agreement between the employer and the employee

10. Hepatitis _____ and _____ are blood borne diseases that that can cause death

11. Handling _____ is hard for most people

12. Ask for _____ when receiving constructive criticism

13. _____ requires that each state keep a registry of nursing assistants

14. The federal government requires that nursing assistants have _____ of continuing education

15. _____ is a state of being frightened , excited, confused, in danger or irritated

16. Something that causes stress is a _____

17. Your_____ of stress depends on your personality, life experiences and physical health

18. _____ groups can help you deal with different types of stress

19. Be _____ of the work you have chosen to do. It is important

20. Exercise _____ is one way to decrease stress

21. _____ health educators and prevention professionals teach the general population or specific populations

22. Searching the _____ is one good way to find a job

23. Be _____ and make eye contact while interviewing

24. Hostile criticism and _____ criticism are not the same thing

25. Constructive criticism is meant to help you _____

ANSWERS

SECTION ONE

1. A

2. C

3. A

4. True

5. A

6. C

7. B

8. B

9. C

10. B

11. A

12. C

13. A

14. True

15. False

16. B

17. C

18. True

19. B

20. B

SECTION TWO

1. J

2. I

3. H

4. G

5. F

6. E

7. D

8. C

9. B

10. A

11. A

12. True

13. B

14. H

15. G

16. F

17. E

18. D

19. C

20. B

21. A

22. D

23. True

24. A

25. D

26. C

27. B

28. A

29. F

30. E

SECTION THREE

1. C

2. A

3. True

4. B

5. B

6. D

7. B

8. C

9. M

10. L

11. K

12. J

13. I

14. H

15. G

16. F

17. E

18. D

19. C

20. A

21. B

22. C

23. C

24. B

25. True

SECTION FOUR

1. C

2. A

3. True

4. True

5. B

6. B

7. A

8. D

9. A

10. True

11. C

12. A

13. D

14. B

15. B

16. C

17. C

18. D

19. A

20. F

21. E

22. D

23. C

24. B

25. A

SECTION FIVE

1. C

2. B

3. A

4. True

5. C

6. B

7. A

8. A

9. B

10. B

11. D

12. C

13. B

14. A

15. D

16. True

17. B

18. C

19. C

20. A

21. D

22. B

23. A

24. C

25. C

SECTION SIX

1. D

2. B

3. True

4. A

5. C

6. B

7. B

8. False

9. A

10. True

11. D

12. True

13. A

14. C

15. C

16. D

17. A

18. True

19. C

20. False

21. A

22. True

23. B

24. True

25. True

SECTION SEVEN

1. C

2. A

3. B

4. D

5. A

6. B

7. D

8. C

9. A

10. B

11. D

12. D

13. C

14. B

15. A

16. D

17. C

18. B

19. A

20. C

21. B

22. D

23. A

24. C

25. D

SECTION EIGHT

1. D

2. A

3. C

4. D

5. B

6. D

7. A

8. A

9. Buddhism

10. Christianity

11. Hinduism

12. Islam

13. Atheists

14. Juduism

15. C

16. B

17. D

18. A

19. C

20. C

21. B

22. D

23. A

24. A

25. C

SECTION NINE

1. A

2. C

3. D

4. B

5. B

6. A

7. D

8. C

9. A

10. D

11. B

12. D

13. C

14. D

15. A

16. B

17. C

18. C

19. A

20. D

21. D

22. A

23. C

24. B

25. B

SECTION TEN

1. A

2. C

3. B

4. A

5. C

6. True

7. A

8. C

9. B

10. B

11. A

12. B

13. C

14. B

15. B

16. A

17. C

18. A

19. B

20. A

21. A

22. C

23. B

24. A

25. C

SECTION ELEVEN

1. Arrives

2. Bed, tidy

3. Admission kit

4. Time, condition

5. Consciousness, confused

6. Introduce, position

7. Friendly

8. Formal

9. Resident

10. Welcome, wanted

11. Tour

12. Valuables

13. Wants, them

14. True

15. True

16. False

17. True

18. False

19. False

20. True

21. False

22. True

23. True

24. False

25. False

SECTION TWELVE

1. True

2. True

3. False

4. False

5. True

6. False

7. False

8. True

9. False

10. False

11. True

12. True

13. True

14. False

15. False

16. False

17. False

18. True

19. True

20. True

21. False

22. True

23. False

24. False

25. True

SECTION THIRTEEN

1. A

2. B

3. B

4. C

5. D

6. A

7. B

8. C

9. D

10. C

11. B

12. A

13. D

14. A

15. B

16. C

17. D

18. A

19. D

20. B

21. C

22. D

23. B

24. C

25. A

SECTION FOURTEEN

1. C

2. A

3. D

4. C

5. B

6. D

7. A

8. C

9. B

10. D

11. A

12. D

13. B

14. C

15. A

16. D

17. C

18. True

19. False

20. True

21. False

22. True

23. False

24. True

25. False

SECTION FIFTEEN

1. B

2. D

3. A

4. B

5. C

6. A

7. D

8. B

9. C

10. A

11. True

12. True

13. False

14. False

15. False

16. True

17. True

18. F

19. H

20. E

21. G

22. A

23. B

24. C

25. D

SECTION SIXTEEN

1. C

2. D

3. B

4. A

5. D

6. C

7. B

8. A

9. C

10. B

11. D

12. True

13. False

14. False

15. False

16. False

17. True

18. True

19. True

20. True

21. False

22. True

23. True

24. False

25. False

SECTION SEVENTEEN

1. True

2. True

3. False

4. True

5. True

6. True

7. False

8. False

9. Enema

10. Fecal impaction

11. Hemorrhoids

12. Diarrhea

13. Flatus or gas

14. Lactose intolerance

15. BRAT

16. Colitis

17. Malabsorption

18. Harris flush

19. Weakening

20. Peptic ulcers

21. Colon cancer

22. 120 ml

23. Blood

24. Worms and amoebas

25. Occult

SECTION EIGHTEEN

1. Sarcoptes scabiei

2. Shingles

3. Wound

4. Inflammation

5. Itching

6. Ringworm

7. Autoimmune illness

8. Women

9. Closed

10. Muscular dystrophy (MD)

11. Amputation

12. Complimentary medicine

13. CVA

14. Right

15. Parkinson

16. Circulation

17. Impairments

18. Spinal cord

19. Safe

20. Glaucoma

21. Atherosclerosis

22. Angina pectoris

23. Myocardial infarction

24. Hyperthyroidism

25. Vaginitis

SECTION NINETEEN

1. F

2. I

3. G

4. H

5. E

6. D

7. B

8. C

9. A

10. A

11. D

12. B

13. A

14. B

15. B

16. C

17. B

18. D

19. B

20. A

21. A

22. C

23. D

24. C

25. D

SECTION TWENTY

1. V

2. U

3. T

4. S

5. R

6. Q

7. P

8. O

9. N

10. M

11. K

12. L

13. H

14. F

15. E

16. D

17. J

18. I

19. G

20. C

21. B

22. A

23. A

24. D

25. B

SECTION TWENTY ONE

1. L

2. H

3. F

4. O

5. A

6. B

7. N

8. C

9. D

10. E

11. G

12. I

13. J

14. M

15. K

16. Rehabilitation

17. Physical and mental health

18. High blood pressure

19. Lower

20. Plate guard

21. Trapeze

22. Belts, cuffs or suction

23. Increase circulation

24. Lungs

25. Incentive spirometers

SECTION TWENTY TWO

1. True

2. True

3. False

4. False

5. True

6. False

7. False

8. False

9. True

10. True

11. True

12. False

13. True

14. Tracheostomy

15. Mechanical ventilation

16. Larynx

17. Sedative

18. Mucus, secretions

19. Chest tubes

20. Pleural cavity

21. Compassionate

22. Constipation

23. Membrane, covers, protects

24. Nostrils flaring

25. Doctor

SECTION TWENTY THREE

1. C

2. A

3. B

4. D

5. A

6. D

7. B

8. C

9. A

10. H

11. K

12. J

13. I

14. G

15. A

16. B

17. C

18. D

19. E

20. F

21. True

22. True

23. True

24. False

25. True

SECTION TWENTY FOUR

1. Direct service

2. Lab technicians

3. Hands-on

4. Potential

5. Called

6. Resume

7. Lie

8. Criminal

9. Job description

10. B and C

11. Criticism

12. Suggestions

13. OBRA

14. 12 hours

15. Stress

16. Stressor

17. Tolerance

18. Support

19. Proud

20. Regularly

21. Health

22. Internet

23. Polite

24. Constructive

25. Improve

SECTION TWENTY FIVE

1. Mucus from the respiratory system that is expectorated from the mouth is called:

   A. Hemoptysis
   B. Acetone
   C. Melena
   D. Sputum

2. Specimens are collected and tested for the following reasons except:

   A. To prevent disease
   B. To detect disease
   C. For urine control
   D. To treat disease

3. Who orders what specimen to collect and the test needed?

   A. Nurse Aide
   B. Doctor
   C. Receptionist
   D. Resident's family

4. Which one is a not rule for collecting specimens?

   A. Use only one container for different specimen
   B. Follow the rules of medical asepsis
   C. Label the container
   D. Do not touch the inside of the container or lid.

5. Urine specimens are collected for:
   A. Tarry stool test
   B. Sputum
   C. Blood test
   D. Urine tests

6. Before collecting a urine specimen you need the following information from the nurse except:

   A. The type of specimen needed
   B. What time to collect the specimen?
   C. How the lab will test the specimen

D. What special measures are needed?

7. The midstream specimen is called_____

    A. A sterile voided specimen
    B. A clean-voided specimen
    C. Acetone specimen
    D. Ketone specimen

8. All urine voided during a 24 hour period is collected for _____.

    A. 24 hour urine specimen
    B. 12 hour urine specimen
    C. Double voided specimen
    D. Random specimen

9. Urine tested for ketones are usually collected:

    A. Before breakfast
    B. Thirty minutes after meals and at bed time
    C. Thirty minutes before meals and at bed time
    D. At midnight

10. Stools are black and tarry if there is bleeding in the:

    A. Intestine
    B. Vagina
    C. Heart
    D. Stomach or upper GI tract.

11. Surgery done by choice to improve the person's life or well-being is called:
    A. Urgent surgery
    B. Emergency surgery
    C. Elective surgery
    D. General surgery

12. Joint replacement surgery and cosmetic surgery are what type of surgery?

    A. General surgery
    B. Elective surgery
    C. Emergency surgery
    D. Urgent surgery

13. The type of surgery that is sudden and unexpected is _____.

   A. Emergency surgery
   B. By-pass surgery
   C. General surgery
   D. Urgent surgery

14. The introduction of fluid into vagina and the immediate return of the fluid is called:

   A. Anesthesia
   B. Thrombus
   C. Embolus
   D. Douche

15. Which is not common fear and concerns of surgical patients?

   A. Pain during surgery
   B. Dying during surgery
   C. Comfort after surgery
   D. Waking up during surgery

16. Regional anesthesia mean:

   A. Loss of consciousness and all feeling
   B. Loss of feeling or sensation in a large area of the body
   C. Loss of feeling or sensation produced by a drug
   D. Loss of feeling or sensation produced by a drug

17. Preoperative drugs are given to patients about _____ minutes to I hour before surgery.

   A. 45
   B. 30
   C. 48
   D. 20

18. Preoperative drugs are given to the patient for the following reasons except:

   A. To help the person relax an feel drowsy
   B. To stop the person from dying
   C. Reduce respirations, secretions and to prevent aspirations.
   D. To prevent nausea and vomiting

19. A doctor who specializes in giving anesthetics is called:

   A. Podiatrist
   B. Social Worker
   C. Physical therapist
   D. An anesthesiologist

20. As CNA to help prevent respiratory and circulatory complications after surgery, you should reposition the patient at
   least:

   A. 96h
   B. q4h
   C. q2h
   D. q3h

21. When preparing surgical patient bed, you should do the following except:

   A. Make a surgical bed
   B. Keep the bed to its lowest position
   C. Lower bed rails
   D. Move furniture out of the way for stretcher

22. Elastic stockings are ordered for the people at risk of thrombi. Which patient is not at risk of thrombi?

   A. Pregnant women
   B. Obese patients
   C. Surgical Patients
   D. None of the above

23. Elastic stocking are also called:

   A. Leg wear
   B. Elastic bandages
   C. Anti-embolism stockings
   D. Pressure stockings

24. Preoperatively Mr. Leon is _____.

   A. Given a tube feeding
   B. NPO

C. Allowed only milk
D. Allowed only water

CIRCLE T IF THE STATEMENT IS TRUE AND F IF IT IS FALSE:

25. The goal of preoperative cane is to prevent complications before, during and after surgery.
T F

26. Surgery is done to remove a diseased body part or repair injured tissue. T F

27. Surgery often requires a hospital stay. T F

28. Women can wear artificial nails to surgery. T F

29. Turning and repositioning re done every 3 to 4 hours after surgery. T F

30. An anesthetist is an RN with advanced study giving anesthetics. T F

31. Artificial eyes and artificial limbs are removed before surgery. T F

32. Some surgeries require certain positions. T F

33. A surgical cap keeps hair out of the face and operative site. T F

34. Jewelries are worn to the operating room. T F

35. A full bladder can cause discomfort during a douche. T F

36. An open wound on the lower leg and feet caused by decreased blood flow through the arteries or veins is:

   A. Arterial Ulcer
   B. Decubitus ulcer
   C. Circulatory ulcer
   D. Pressure ulcer

37. Thin watery drainage that is blood-tinged is called:

   A. Sanguineous drainage
   B. Purulent drainage
   C. Serious drainage
   D. Serosanguineos drainage

38. Which is not a type of wound?

    A. Abrasion
    B. Gangrene
    C. Laceration
    D. Contusion

39. Partial-thickness wound caused by the scraping away or rubbing of skin is called:

    A. Incision
    B. Puncture wound
    C. Abrasion
    D. Penetrating wound

40. Violent act that injures the skin, mucous membranes, bones and internal organs is :

    A. Trauma
    B. Wound
    C. Shock
    D. Skin tear

41. Tissues are injured but she skin is not broken. This is called what?

    A. Clean wound
    B. Closed wound
    C. Contaminated wound
    D. Puncture wound

42. Dehiscence means:

    A. Infected wound
    B. Wounds with large amount of microbes
    C. Wounds that does not heal easily
    D. Separation of wound layers

43. A pressure ulcer can also be called:

    A. Decubitus ulcer
    B. Vascular ulcer
    C. Venous ulcer
    D. Chronic ulcer

44. An area where the bone sticks out or projects out from the flat surface of the body is called?

   A. Bedsore
   B. Pressure sore
   C. A bony prominence
   D. Contusion

45. Which one is not a bony prominence?

   A. Shoulder blades
   B. Sacrum
   C. Ankles
   D. Ear

46. Common causes of skin breakdown and pressure ulcers include the following except:

   A. Friction
   B. Shock
   C. Shearing
   D. Pressure

47. The bony areas are called:

   A. Bed sore
   B. Pressure sore
   C. Pressure points
   D. Pressure stage

48. At the first stage of the pressure ulcers the skin is _____.

   A. Cyanosis
   B. Red
   C. Peels
   D. Cracks

49. Which is not measures in preventing pressure ulcers?

   A. Positioning the person according to the care plan
   B. Raising the head of the bed to highest position
   C. Providing good skin care
   D. Minimizing skin exposure to moisture

50. Measures to prevent circulatory ulcers includes the following except:
    A. Keeping pressure of the heels and other bony areas
    B. Do not massage over pressure points
    C. Keeping linens clean, dry and wrinkle free
    D. Dressing the person in tight clothes

51. Heat and cold application for promoting healing and comfort is ordered by:

    A. Doctor
    B. Nurse
    C. CNA
    D. Receptionist

52. Bluish skin color is _____-.

    A. Syncope
    B. Erythema
    C. Jaundice
    D. Cyanosis

53. A body temperature is much larger than the person's normal. This is called:

    A. Hypothermia
    B. Hyperthermia
    C. Low blood pressure
    D. Blood pressure rate

54. Heat applications are often used for:

    A. Circulatory problems
    B. Musculoskeletal injuries
    C. Nervous Injuries
    D. Heart Injuries

55. Which is not a reason for heat application?

    A. To relieve Pain
    B. To increase joint stiffness
    C. To reduce tissue swelling
    D. To relaxes muscles

56. What type of application has greater and fasten effects:

   A. Dry heat application
   B. Non-dry application
   C. Heat application
   D. Moist heat application

57. A cold application is usually between:

   A. 50° to 65° F
   B. 98° to 106° F
   C. 100° to 106° F
   D. 40° to 50° F

58. Heat and cold are applied for not longer than:

   A. 2 to 5 minutes
   B. 5 to 10 minutes
   C. 15 to 20 minutes
   D. 10 to 15 minutes

59. A very hot application is apply only by:

   A. Charge Nurse
   B. Nursing assistant
   C. Physical therapist
   D. Occupational therapist

60. Very hot application is usually between:

   A. 95° to 108° F
   B. 106° to 120° F
   C. 105° to 106° F
   D. 106° to 115° F

61. The Sitz bath usually last for:

   A. 5 minutes
   B. 20 minutes
   C. 45 minutes

D. 50 minutes

62. An electric device used for dry heat is:

    A. Compress
    B. Compass
    C. The aquachermia pad
    D. Hypothermia pad

63. Which one is not a sign and symptom of hypoxia?

    A. Dizziness
    B. Confusion
    C. Rash
    D. Fatigue

64. Hypoxia means _____.

    A. Rapid breathing
    B. Insufficient oxygen to the cells
    C. Slow breathing
    D. Abnormal breathing

65. Smoking causes:

    A. Lung cancer
    B. Breath cancer
    C. Kidney failure
    D. Heart Cancer

66. An early sign of hypoxia is:

    A. Apprehension
    B. Agitation
    C. Cyanosis
    D. Restlessness

67. Breathing deeply and comfortably only when sitting is called:

    A. Dyspnea
    B. Orthopnea
    C. Apnea
    D. Bradypnea

68. Slow, weak respirations at not fewer than 12 per minute is:

    A. Cheyenne-strokes respirations
    B. Biot's respiration
    C. Respiratory depression
    D. Respiratory arrest

69. Pulmonary function test measures:

    A. The amount of oxygen in the blood
    B. The amount of hemoglobin containing oxygen
    C. The amount of air moving in and out of the lungs
    D. How much air the heart can hold

70. A chest X-ray is taken to detect:

    A. Blood damage
    B. Lung damage
    C. Kidney damage
    D. Liver damage

71. A substance that gives off radiation is called:

    A. Bronchoscopy
    B. Thoracentesis
    C. Radiation
    D. Radioisotope

72. Pulse oximetry measures:

    A. Oxygen concentration in arterial blood
    B. The amount of brain damage
    C. The capacity of air the lungs can hold
    D. Measures progress of lungs disease.

73. Breathing is usually easier in what type of position?

    A. Sims's position
    B. Prone position
    C. Fowler's Position
    D. Supine position

74. Factors affecting oxygen needs include:

    A. Respiratory system status
    B. Aging
    C. Pain
    D. All of the above

75. People with difficulty breathing often prefer sitting-up and leaning over a table to breathe. This is called:

    A. Dorsal Recumbent position
    B. Knee-chest position
    C. Orthopneic position
    D. Lithotomy position

76. Position changes are needed at least for:

    A. q6h
    B. q2h
    C. q3h
    D. q8h

77. You are assisting a patient with coughing and deep breathing. Which is incorrect?

    A. The person inhales through pursed lips
    B. The person sits on comfortable position
    C. The person holds a follow over air incision
    D. The person inhales deeply through the nose

78. The collapse of a portion of the lungs is called:

    A. Pneumonia
    B. Dizziness
    C. Atelectasis
    D. Disorientation

79. A spirometer is a machine that measures:

    A. The movement of air
    B. The amount of air moving out of the lungs

C. The volume of air exhaled

D. The amount of air inhaled

80. The amount of oxygen to give and the device to use can only be ordered by _____.

    A. CNA

    B. Doctor

    C. RN

    D. LVN

81. Oropharyngeal airway is inserted through:

    A. Nostril and into the pharynx

    B. Nose and into the trachea

    C. The mouth and into the pharynx

    D. The surgically created opening into the trachea

82. Which one is not the upper part of the airway (Upper respiratory tract)?

    A. Mouth

    B. Pharynx

    C. Mouth

    D. The trachea

83. Infection of the middle ear is called:

    A. Otitis media

    B. Deaf

    C. Cerumen

    D. Braille

84. Otitis media is common in _____.

    A. Young people

    B. Old people

    C. Infants

    D. Adults

85. A chronic disease of the inner ear is _____.

    A. Tinnitus

    B. Otitis media

    C. Acute Ear Disease

D. Meniere's Disease

86. The middle ear contains Eustachian tube and three small bones called:

   A. Eardrum
   B. Tympanic membrane
   C. Ossicles
   D. Auditory canal

87. Difficulty in hearing normal conversation is _____.

   A. Deafness
   B. Hearing loss
   C. Vertigo
   D. Cerumen

88. Hearing loss in which is impossible for the person to understand speech through hearing alone is _____.

   A. Hearing loss
   B. Deafness
   C. Tinnitus
   D. Otitis media

89. The most common cause of hearing loss in children is

   A. Illness
   B. Birth defects
   C. Ear infection
   D. Injury

90. Symptoms of hearing loss in children and adult include:

   A. Speaking too loudly
   B. Leaning forward to hear
   C. Asking for words to be repeated
   D. All of the above

91. Communicating with hearing impaired person includes the following except:

   A. Position yourself at the person's level
   B. Turn your back when speaking with the person

C. Stand or sit in good right.
D. Speak clearly, distinctly and slowly

92. The second layer of the eyes is called:

   A. The sclera
   B. The retina
   C. The Choroid layer
   D. Optic nerve

93. The major cause of vision loss is _____.

   A. Cataract
   B. Infections
   C. Glaucoma
   D. Hereditary

94. Hearing aids make:

   A. Sounds louder
   B. Speech clearer
   C. Correct hearing disorder
   D. Increase background noise

95. Braille involves:

   A. Ringing in the ears
   B. Raise dots arrange for letters of the alphabet
   C. Dizziness
   D. Audio Books

96. CNA can provide safety for blind clients by doing the following except:

   A. Turning on lights
   B. Keeping doors open or closed
   C. Having client stand in the middle of room
   D. Informing the client of steps and curbs

97. When communicating with the speech impaired, you should do the following
   A. Listen, and give the person full attention
   B. Determine the subject been discussed
   C. Repeat what the person has said
   D. All of the above

98. _____ is a disease affecting the blood vessels that supply blood to the brain.

   A. Angina pectoris
   B. Myocardial infarction
   C. Stroke
   D. Heart attack

99. The third leading cause of death in the United States is _____.

   A. Heart attack
   B. Cerebrovascular accident
   C. Diabetes
   D. Obesity

100. The surgical creation of an artificial opening between the ureter and the abdomen is called:

   A. Ureterostomy
   B. Ileostomy
   C. Bosomy
   D. Colostomy

101. High sugar in the blood is called:

   A. Hypoglycemia
   B. Diabetes mellitus
   C. Sugar Surge
   D. Hyperglycemia

102. _____ is a tumor that grows fast and invades other tissues.

   A. Fast tumor
   B. Malign tumor
   C. Benign tumor
   D. Metastasis

103. The removal of all or part of an extremity is _____.

   A. Amputation
   B. Decapitation
   C. Evisceration
   D. Cutting

104. Which therapy helps the immune system?

A. Hormone therapy
B. Chemotherapy
C. Biological therapy
D. Radiation therapy

105. The followings are the side effect of hormone therapy except:

A. Weight gain
B. Fatigue
C. Hot flashes
D. Muscle aches

106. Leukemia is the most common type of _____ in children.

A. Myocardial infarction
B. Cancer
C. Pneumonia
D. Stroke

107. Which of the followings can be a care for people with paralysis?

A. Keep the bed in low position
B. Follow bowel and bladder training programs
C. Maintain good alignment at all times.
D. All of the above.

108. _____ is spread by airborne droplets with coughing, sneezing, speaking, and singing.

A. Pneumonia
B. Leprosy
C. Asthma
D. Tuberculosis

109. The leading cause of death In United States is _____.

A. Coronary Artery Disease
B. Pneumonia
C. HIV
D. Angina

110. Which of the followings is the major complication of CAD?

   A. Emphysema
   B. Dyspnea
   C. Tuberculosis
   D. Myocardial infarction

111. _____ occurs when the heart cannot pump blood normally.

   A. Hypertension
   B. Congestive heart failure
   C. Hypotension
   D. None of the above

112. Blood clot is also known as _____.

   A. Bronchus
   B. Thrombus
   C. Blood stop
   D. Platelets

113. The therapy that involves drugs that kill cells is called:

   A. Hormone therapy
   B. Biological therapy
   C. Chemotherapy
   D. Physiotherapy

114. Using X-ray beams to destroy cancerous cells is _____ therapy.

   A. Radiotherapy
   B. Physiotherapy
   C. Chemotherapy
   D. Biological therapy

115. _____ is the spread of cancer to other parts of the body.

   A. Stomatitis
   B. Cancer transfer
   C. Benign tumor
   D. Metastasis

116. A condition in which there is death of tissue is called:

    A. Aphasia
    B. Gangrene
    C. Angina
    D. Pectoris

117. _____ is when the bone becomes porous and brittle or is fragile and breaks easily.

    A. Osteoporosis
    B. Arthritis
    C. Rheumatoid arthritis
    D. Bone low density

118. Which of the followings is not a rule for cast care?

    A. Turn the person every two hours
    B. Wash the cast every 4hours
    C. Elevate a casted arm or leg on pillows
    D. Protect the person from rough cast edges.

119. Which of the followings is not a risk factor of stroke?

    A. Smoking
    B. Obesity
    C. Exercise
    D. Drug abuse

120. There ___ major types of hepatitis.

    A. 5
    B. 3
    C. 6
    D. 4

121. Diseases that are contagious and infectious are called_____ diseases.

    A. Non-communicable
    B. Spreading
    C. Communicable
    D. Rapid

122. Which one is a sign and symptom of hepatitis?

   A. Loss of appetite
   B. Fever
   C. Nausea and vomiting
   D. All of the above

123. What type of diabetes occurs mostly in children?

   A. Type 2
   B. Type 3
   C. Type 1
   D. Type 4

124. Which of these is a sign of chronic renal failure?

   A. Sudden severe headaches with no known cause
   B. Halitosis
   C. Rashes
   D. Rigidity and trembling of extremities

125. The pathway created for urine to exit the body by removing the bladder is called _____.

   A. Urinary Diversion
   B. Urinary conversion
   C. Urinary obstruction
   D. Urinary bisection

126. Cystitis which is a bladder infection is caused by _____.

   A. Virus
   B. Fungus
   C. Bacteria
   D. Nematode

127. Care of a person with stroke involves the following except:

   A. The bed is kept in semi-Fowler's position
   B. Avoid coughing and deep breathing.
   C. Food and fluids needs are met
   D. Good skin care prevents pressure ulcers

128. Psychosis means:

A. A state of severe mental impairment
B. A disorder of the mind
C. Mental disorder
D. Emotional illness

129. Superego is concerned with_____.

A. Ability and disability
B. Mind and stress
C. Right and wrong
D. Health and illness

130. A vague uneasy feeling in response to stress is called:

A. Personality
B. Anxiety
C. Stress
D. Panic

131. Which one is not a sign and symptom of anxiety?

A. Rapid pulse
B. Rapid respiration
C. Increased blood pressure
D. Redness

132. Any factor that causes stress is called:

A. Obsession
B. Stress
C. A stressor
D. Phobia

133. The highest level of anxiety is _____.

A. Syncope
B. Panic
C. Dread
D. Terror

134. Which is not a sign and symptom of depression in older people?

   A. Diarrhea
   B. Paranoia
   C. Dry mouth
   D. Anxiety

135. Depression involves the following except:

   A. Body
   B. Mood
   C. Ability
   D. Thoughts

136. _____ when a person is seeing, hearing or feeling something that is not real.

   A. Delusion
   B. Hallucination
   C. Paranoia
   D. Bipolar disorder

137. Mrs. White believes that she is the Queen of England. This is called a _____.

   A. Hallucination
   B. Paranoia
   C. Delusion of persecution
   D. Delusion of grandeur

138. Mr. Smith believes that his food is poisoned. This is called a _____.

   A. Superego
   B. Paranoia
   C. Psychosis
   D. Delusion

139. Anorexia nervosa occurs when?

   A. A person has an intense fear of weight gain and obesity
   B. Binge eating occurs
   C. A person explore his or her thoughts and feelings
   D. A person has severe extremes in mood

140. Repeating an act over and again without the ability to control the repetition is called:

A. Ego

B. Paraphrasing

C. Compulsion

D. Conscious

141. Delirium means:

A. A false belief

B. Loss of conjecture and social function

C. Feeling something that is not real

D. A state of temporary but acute mental confusion

142. Cognitive functioning includes all except:

A. Memory

B. Attitude

C. Thinking

D. Reasoning

143. When caring for a confused person the CNA should do the following except:

A. Provide safety

B. Give date and time each morning

C. Rearrange Furniture and the person's view

D. Place familiar objects and pictures within the person's view

144. Loss of cognitive and social function caused by changes in the brain is called

A. Dementia

B. Paranoia

C. Obsession

D. Schizophrenia

145. Alzheimer's disease is:

A. Heart disease

B. Brain disease

C. Blood disease

D. Liver disease

146. The most common type of permanent dementia is _____.

A. Huntington's disease
B. Parkinson's disease
C. Alzheimer's disease
D. Korsakoff disease

147. The most common mental health problem in old people is

A. Depression
B. Infection
C. Drugs
D. Head injuries

148. Signs and symptoms of delirium include:

A. Tremors
B. Delusions
C. Hallucinations
D. All of the above

149. Mr. Fresh has delusion. Delusion means:

A. False dementia
B. False belief
C. A state of Temporary but acute mental confusion
D. Something that is not real

150. Signs, symptoms and behavior of Alzheimer's disease increase during:

A. Daylight
B. Morning time
C. Early afternoon
D. Hours of dark

151. The classic sign of Alzheimer's disease is _____-.

A. Not recognizing objects
B. Gradual loss of short term memory
C. Agitation
D. Mood and personality

152. The followings are common in people with Alzheimer's disease except

A. Pain, rash and shock

B. Communication problem, moodiness and restlessness
C. Memory loss, poor judgment and poor reasoning
D. Delusion, hallucination and screaming

153. When caring for Mr. Stone who is wandering you should do the following except:

A. Follow agency policy for locking doors and windows
B. Keep door alarms and electronic doors turned on
C. Involve the person with activities
D. Restraint Mr. Stone firmly

154. Mr. Jones becomes confused and begins to wander. The CNA should:

A. Restrain him to prevent injuries
B. Tell the doctor
C. Report his behavior to the charge nurse
D. Tell his family about the behavior

155. A common sign of depression is:
A. Laughing and smiling
B. Changes in appetite
C. Socializing with friends
D. Attending activities

156. a disability occurring before 22years of age is called a _____.

A. Developmental disability
B. Mental retardation
C. Spastic
D. Spinal bifida

157. Mental retardation involves:

A. Violent sudden contractions of muscle groups
B. Muscle weakness
C. Low intellectual function
D. Uncontrolled contraction of skeletal muscles

158. These statements are about cerebral palsy. Which one is false?

A. It is a disorder involving muscle weakness or poor muscle
B. It is violent contractions of muscle group
C. Lack of oxygen to the brain is the usual cause

D. The defect is in the motor region of the brain

159. Autism begins in early childhood between:

A. 12months and six years
B. 9 months and 7years
C. 10 months and 5years
D. 18 months and 3years

160. Paralysis of all four extremities is:

A. Paraplegia
B. Hemiplegia
C. Quadriplegia
D. Diplegia

161. Paralysis of one side of the body is

A. Quadriplegia
B. Hemiplegia
C. Paraplegia
D. Diplegia

162. Diplegia means:

A. That similar body part are affected on both side of the body
B. The arm and leg on one side are affected
C. Both arms and both legs are paralyzed so are the trunks and neck muscles.
D. Paralysis of the leg or lower body

163. People with cerebral palsy have much impairment. They include the following except:

A. Mental retardation
B. Learning disabilities
C. Speech impairments
D. Wide flat nose

164. A chronic conditions produced by temporary changes in the brains electrical function is:

A. Autism
B. Epilepsy
C. Spina bifida
D. Hydrocephalus

165. Seizures that occur in one part of the brain is called:

A. Whole seizures
B. Single seizures
C. Partial seizures
D. Generalized seizures

166. Spina bifida defects occur during the:

A. 3 months of pregnancy
B. First month of pregnancy
C. 6 months of pregnancy
D. 5 months of pregnancy

167. Down syndrome occurs:

A. First month of pregnancy
B. At fertilization
C. During birth
D. From trauma

168. Children with Down syndrome has certain features caused by extra chromosomes. They include the following
   Except:

A. Drooling
B. Over shaped eyes that slant upwards
C. Flat face
D. Short, wide hands with stubby fingers

169. A seizure can also be called:

A. Autism
B. Down syndrome
C. Convulsion
D. Spina bifida

170. Spina bifida involves...............

A. Loss of consciousness
B. A defect of spinal column

C. Hearing impairments

D. Mental retardation

171. The inability of the male to have an erection is called:

A. Menopause

B. Impotence

C. Transvestite

D. Transsexual

172. Erectile dysfunction is same thing as:

A. Impotence

B. Menopause

C. Bisexual

D. Transsexual

173. Menopause is _____.

A. When the body responds to stimulation

B. When menstruation stops

C. Reproduce organ

D. Uniting of the sperm and ovum

174. Menstruation occurs about every:

A. 20 days

B. 18 days

C. 10 days

D. 28 days

175. Menopause occurs between _____ and _____ years of age.

A. 30 and 40

B. 30 and 35

C. 45 and 55

D. 50 and 60

CIRCLE T IF THE STATEMENT IS TRUE AND F IF IT IS FALSE.

176. Reproductive organs change with aging. T F

177. Diabetes and spinal cord injuries can cause impotence. T F

178. Heterosexual is a person who is attracted to both sexes. T F

179. Sexuality is important to small children. T F

180. Injury, Illness and surgery can affect sexual function. T F

181. Lochia means:

   A. Person feelings and attitudes about his or her sex
   B. Surgical removal of foreskin from the penis
   C. Vaginal discharge that occurs after child birth.
   D. Incision into perineum

182. Signs and symptoms of illness in babies include the followings except:

   A. The body is limp and slow to respond
   B. The body has a low temperature
   C. The bay is flashed, pale or perspiring
   D. The body has reddened or irritated eyes

183. As a CNA you can help with breast feeding in the following ways:

   A. Helping the mother to a comfortable position
   B. Making sure the mother holds the baby close to her breast
   C. Having the mother use her nipple to stroke the baby's cheek or lower lip.
   D. All of the above

184. Breast-fed babies usually nurse every:

   A. 8 or 12 hours
   B. 4 or 8 hours
   C. 2 or 3 hours
   D. 3 or 6 hours

185. Babies are fed on:

   A. Schedule
   B. Demand
   C. All time
   D. On their mother's free time

186. Safety measures for infant includes the following except:

    A. Laying an infant on soft bedding products.
    B. Support the baby's head and neck when lifting or holding the baby
    C. Handle the baby with gentle smooth movements
    D. Use both hands to lift a newborn baby

187. Nursing mother needs:

    A. Spicy and gas forming foods
    B. Caffeine
    C. Cola beverages
    D. Good nutrition

188. Infant birth weight is the baseline for measuring:

    A. Weight
    B. Growth
    C. Height
    D. Amount of milk taken

189. When bathing a new born baby the water temperature should be _____ to _____ degrees F:

    A. 80 to 90
    B. 90 to 95
    C. 100 to 105
    D. 100 to 150

190. Which of the following is used to wash a new born baby's nose?

    A. A mitted wash cloths
    B. Cotton balls
    C. Alcohol swipes
    D. A cotton swab

191. CNA should report the followings to the charge nurse when caring for new born babies except:

    A. The baby has reddened or irritated eyes
    B. The baby spit a small amount when burped
    C. Stools are light-colored
    D. The baby looks flushed, pale and perspiring

192. A baby's head and neck is supported for the first_____ months.

    A. 9
    B. 6
    C. 8
    D. 3

193. When bottle-feeding babies. You should:

    A. Prop the bottle and lay the baby down for the feeding
    B. Force the baby to finish the bottle
    C. Hold the baby close to you
    D. Leave the baby at one inch with the bottle

194. Burping a baby is also called

    A. Breast-feeding
    B. Bubbling
    C. Diapering
    D. Circumcision

195. Newborns usually have a bowel movement with every feeding. T F

196. Watery stools means constipation. T F

197. Baby stops sucking and turns away from the bottle when satisfied. T F

198. You can lift a newborn by the arm. T F

199. Moisture, feces, and urine irritate baby's skin. T F

200. Umbilical cord carries blood, oxygen and nutrients from the mother to fetus. T F

201. A written plan listing the services needed by the person and who provides them is_____.

    A. Meal plan
    B. ADL plan
    C. A service plan
    D. Nursing Services

202. Assisted living provides the following except:

    A. Healthcare
    B. Nursing care
    C. Housing
    D. Support services

203. CNA should report any drug error to:

    A. RN
    B. Co-worker
    C. Receptionist
    D. Doctor

204. Medication records should include the following except:

    A. The person's name
    B. Date of birth of the person
    C. Drug name, dose directions, and route of administration
    D. Date and time to take the drug

205. Which of the following is not drug error?

    A. Taking the wrong dose
    B. Taking another person's drug
    C. Taking a drug when ordered
    D. Taking a drug at the wrong time

206. Drugs are kept in:

    A. Closet
    B. On top of table
    C. Under the bed
    D. IN a locked container, cabinet or area

207. Certain measures are needed when handling, preparing and storing food. It includes the following except:

    A. Empty garbage at least once in two weeks
    B. Protect left over foods
    C. Wash cooking and eating items
    D. Place washed eating and cooking items in a drainer to dry

208. CNA can assist with drugs in the following ways except:

A. Reminding the person it is time to take the drug
B. Giving drugs
C. Reading the drug label to the person
D. Opening containers for people who cannot do so

209. Transfer, discharge and eviction of person can happen for the following reasons:

A. The person fails to pay for services
B. The person wants to transfer
C. The facility closes
D. All of the above

210. Housekeeping measures help prevent infection in the following ways except:

A. Cleaning tub or shower after each use
B. Cleaning bathroom surfaces once in three weeks
C. Dusting furniture at least weekly
D. Vacuum floors at least weekly and as needed

211. When assisting with laundry services you should:

A. Follow your own preferences
B. Wash with hot water
C. Follow care label directions
D. Wash sturdy and delicate fabrics together

212. An assisted living resident is encouraged to eat in:

A. Dining room
B. Inner room
C. Bathroom
D. Kitchen

213. Which statement about assisted living is incorrect?

A. Assisted living provide secured and 24 hour supervision for residents
B. They provide each person with private apartment
C. Three meals a day and snacks are provided
D. They offer social and recreational service

214. Assisted facility residents have the right to:
   A. Be treated with dignity respect, consideration and fairness
   B. Help develop a plan
   C. Receive the services stated in the service plan
   D. All of the above

215. Which is not a requirement and features of assisted living facility units?

   A. A mailbox for each person
   B. A window that allow safe exit in an emergency
   C. A closet with insects and rodents
   D. Smoke detectors

216. The excessive loss of blood in a short time is called:

   A. Blood flow
   B. Blood loss
   C. Hemorrhage
   D. Blood clot

217. _____ occurs when the heart and breathing stop suddenly without warning.

   A. System arrest
   B. Heart malfunction
   C. Cardiac Arrest
   D. Heart stoppage

218. The emergency care given to an ill or injured person before medical help arrives is called:

   A. Initial aid
   B. First aid
   C. Last Aid
   D. Emergency aid

219. When breathing stops but heart action continues for several minutes. This is called:

   A. Respiratory arrest
   B. Heart arrest
   C. Heart seizure
   D. Heart failure

220. To activate EMS system, dial_____

A. 921

B. 112

C. 114

D. 911

221. Which is one of the goals of First Aid?

   A. To cure the person permanently
   B. To prevent injuries from becoming worse
   C. To operate on the patient if the need arises there.
   D. To make sure the person live at all cost

222. Causes of respiratory arrest include the followings except:

   A. Vomiting
   B. Drowning
   C. Smoke inhalation
   D. Suffocation

223. Which of these is not a general rule of emergency care?

   A. Check for life threatening problems
   B. Stay calm
   C. Do not hang up until the operator has hung up
   D. Act with alacrity and temerity

224. The CPR has ____ basic parts.

   A. 2
   B. 4
   C. 3
   D. 5

225. Which of these is not a basic part of CPR?

   A. Smelling
   B. Airway
   C. Breathing
   D. Circulation

226. _____ maneuver opens the airway.

A. Nose tilt
B. Stomach tilt
C. Head-tilt/chin
D. Nose-tilt/chin

227. The AHA's pediatric chain of survival involves these except:

    A. Preventing cardiac arrest and injuries
    B. Later advance care
    C. Early CPR
    D. Early access to emergency response system

228. When practicing CPR, we should use _____.

    A. Babies
    B. Adults
    C. Young people
    D. Mannequins

229. Cardiac arrest caused by heart disease is rare in _____.

    A. Adults
    B. Children
    C. Young people
    D. A and C

230. Which of these can lead to cardiac arrest?

    A. Voiding
    B. FBAO
    C. Vomiting
    D. None of the above

231. A large, poorly chewed piece of meat is a common cause of_____.

    A. Syncope
    B. Dying
    C. Vomiting
    D. FBAO

232. Older people are at risk for choking. Which of these is not a risk?

    A. Strong fitted dentures

B. Poorly fitted dentures
C. Dysphagia
D. Hard candy

233. _____ maneuver is used to relieve FBAO.

   A. Parkinson
   B. Einthoven
   C. Heimlich
   D. Chest

234. _____ results when organs and tissues do not get enough blood.

   A. Syncope
   B. Shock
   C. Convulsion
   D. Cardiac Arrest

235. _____ is violent and sudden contractions or tremors of muscle group.

   A. Shock
   B. Syncope
   C. Heart attack
   D. Convulsion

236. Signs and symptoms of anaphylaxis are the followings except:

   A. Sweating
   B. Shortness of breath
   C. Voiding
   D. Dyspnea

237. Common causes of fires and burns include the following except:

   A. Cautions with matches and lighters
   B. Falling asleep while smoking
   C. Fireplaces
   D. Space heaters

238. _____ is the sudden loss of consciousness from an inadequate blood supply to the brain.

A. Stroke
B. Fainting
C. Cardiac failure
D. Angina pectoris

239. _____ accident occurs when the brain is suddenly deprived of its blood supply.

A. Cardio
B. Reproductive
C. System
D. Cerebrovascular

240. The Heimlich maneuver is performed with people in the following position except:

A. Standing
B. Sitting
C. Walking
D. Lying

241. A document stating a person's wish about healthcare when the person cannot make his or her own decisions is _____.
A. Emergency directives
B. Later directives
C. Advance directives
D. Healthcare directives

242. Post mortem means:

A. During death
B. After Death
C. Before death
D. Death

243. The belief that the spirit or soul is reborn in another body or in another form of life is _____.

A. Resurrection
B. Ascension
C. Awakening
D. Reincarnation

244. There _____ stages of dying.

   A. 5
   B. 3
   C. 4
   D. 7

245. During dying a Mr. John responds and says "NO NOT ME", what dying stage is he in?

   A. Anger
   B. Depression
   C. Denial
   D. Bargaining

246. _____ care focuses on the physical, emotional, social, and spiritual needs of dying people and their families.

   A. Hospital
   B. Hospice
   C. Covalent
   D. Clinic

247. _____ wills is a document about measures that support or maintain life when death is likely.

   A. Person
   B. Living
   C. Dying
   D. Facility

248. The dying person's room should have the following conditions except:

   A. The CNA arrange the room as they wish
   B. The room should be comforting and pleasant
   C. The room should be well lit and well ventilated
   D. The room should reflect the person's choice

249. MRS. Smith is a dying patient and suddenly says "This is not true, I know that I am dreaming…..". Which dying stage is this_____?

   A. Acceptance
   B. Depression

C. Denial

D. Bargaining

250. The dying person bill of right includes the following except:

    A. I have the right to be treated as a living human being till I die

    B. I have the right not to be deceived

    C. I have the right to die with somebody

    D. I have the right to die in peace and dignity

251. Restraints are used only if ordered by _____.

    A. Charge nurse

    B. Doctor

    C. Therapist

    D. CNA

252. When the dying person engages you in conversation. As the CNA you should do the following except:

    A. Let the person express feelings and emotions.

    B. Do not worry about saying the wrong thing or finding comforting words.

    C. Ignore the client

    D. Listen carefully and don't interrupt

253. Dying People often need the following except:

    A. Hospital care

    B. Nursing center

    C. Hospice

    D. Sports center

254. The Stiffness or rigidity of skeletal muscles that occurs after death is called:

    A. Post mortem stiffness

    B. Rigor Mortis

    C. Mortem

    D. Mortis

255. _____ illness or injury for which there is no reasonable expectation of recovery.

    A. Sudden

    B. Emergency

    C. Terminal

    D. Mortem

SECTION TWENTY FIVE ANSWERS

1. D
2. C
3. B
4. A
5. D
6. C
7. B
8. A
9. C
10. D
11. C
12. B
13. A
14. D
15. C
16. B
17. A
18. B
19. D
20. C
21. B
22. D
23. C
24. B
25. T
26. T
27. T
28. F
29. F
30. T
31. T
32. T

33. T
34. F
35. T
36. C
37. D
38. B
39. C
40. A
41. B
42. D
43. A
44. C
45. D
46. B
47. C
48. B
49. B
50. D
51. A
52. D
53. B
54. B
55. B
56. D
57. A
58. C
59. A
60. D
61. B
62. C
63. C
64. B
65. A
66. D
67. B
68. C
69. C
70. B
71. D
72. A
73. C
74. D
75. C

76. B
77. A
78. C
79. D
80. B
81. C
82. D
83. A
84. C
85. D
86. C
87. D
88. A
89. C
90. D
91. B
92. C
93. C
94. A
95. B
96. C
97. D
98. C
99. B
100. A
101. D
102. B
103. A
104. C
105. D
106. B
107. D
108. D
109. A
110. D
111. B
112. B
113. C
114. A
115. D
116. B
117. A

118. B
119. C
120. A
121. C
122. D
123. C
124. B
125. A
126. C
127. B
128. A
129. C
130. B
131. D
132. C
133. B
134. A
135. C
136. B
137. D
138. B
139. A
140. C
141. D
142. B
143. C
144. A
145. B
146. C
147. A
148. D
149. B
150. D
151. B
152. A
153. D
154. C
155. B

156. A
157. C
158. B

159. D
160. C
161. B
162. A
163. D
164. B
165. C
166. B
167. B
168. A
169. C
170. B
171. B
172. A
173. B
174. D
175. C
176. T
177. T
178. F
179. F
180. T
181. C
182. B
183. D
184. C
185. B
186. A
187. D
188. B
189. C
190. A
191. B
192. D
193. C
194. B
195. T
196. F
197. T
198. F
199. T
200. T

201. C
202. B
203. A
204. B
205. C
206. D
207. A
208. B
209. D
210. B
211. C
212. A
213. B
214. D
215. C
216. C
217. C
218. B
219. A
220. D
221. B
222. A
223. D
224. C
225. A
226. C
227. B
228. D
229. B
230. B
231. D
232. A
233. C
234. B
235. D
236. C
237. A
238. B
239. D
240. C
241. C
242. B
243. D

244. A
245. C
246. B
247. B
248. A
249. C
250. C
251. B
252. C
253. D
254. B
255. C

OTHER TITLES FROM THE SAME AUTHOR:

1. Work At Home Jobs For Nurses & Other Healthcare Professionals

2. Nurses' Romance Series

3. BLS for Healthcare Providers Student Manual

4. Patient Care Technician Exam Review Questions: PCT Test Prep

5. Accept Challenges

6. EKG Technician Study guide

7. EKG Test Prep

8. Phlebotomy Test Prep Vol 1, 2, & 3

9. The Home Health Aide Textbook

10. CNA Exam Prep Volume One & Two

And Many More Books

Visit www.janejohn-nwankwo.com

www.bookaspeakernow.com

www.healthcarepracticetest.com

www.djngbooks.org

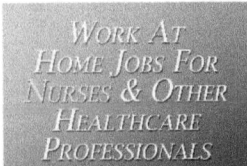
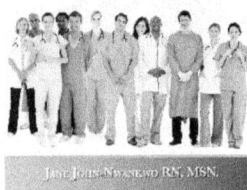
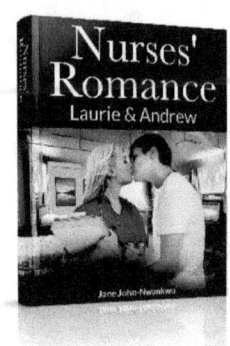
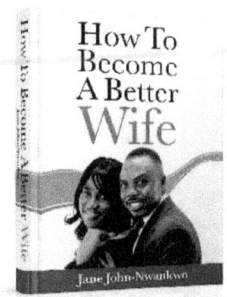
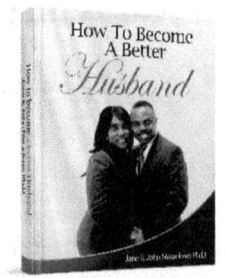

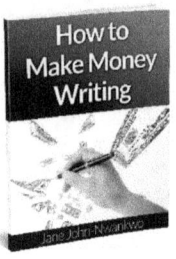
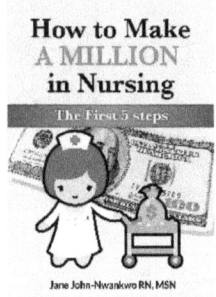
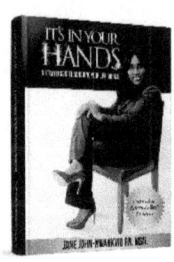
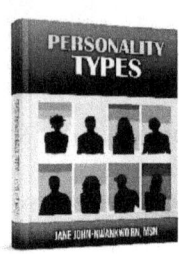

Purchase these books at www.djngbooks.org   **www.janejohn-nwankwo.com**

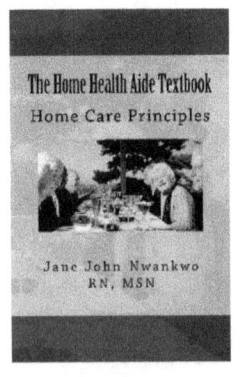
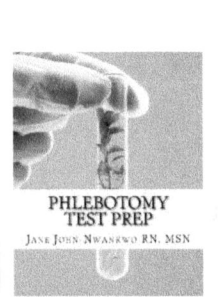
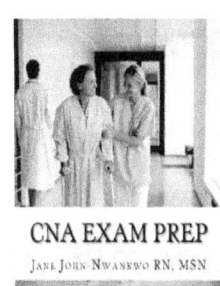
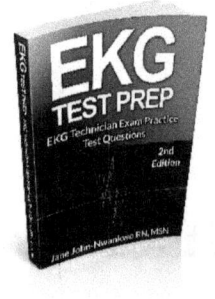
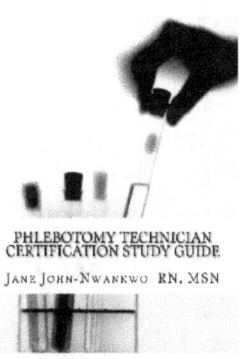

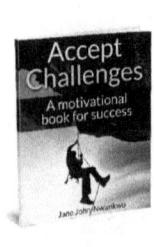
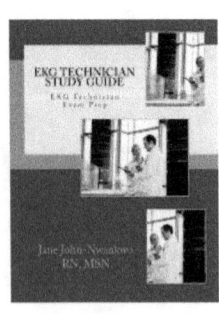
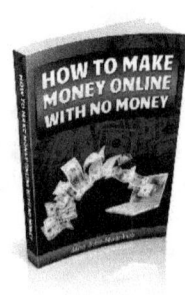
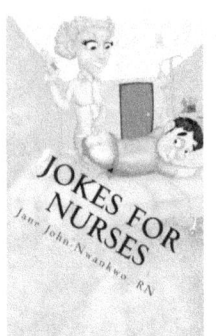
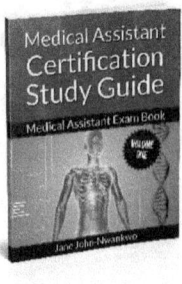

Purchase these books at www.janejohn-nwankwo.com   **www.djngbooks.org**

www.ingramcontent.com/pod-product-compliance
Lightning Source LLC
Chambersburg PA
CBHW080250180526
45167CB00006B/2476